"This wonderful anthology is a feast of a book. ~~myself~~ myself invited, engaged, stimulated, conversed with. Hargaden combines theory, poetry, neurobiology and political thought and weaves them in and out of rich and exciting case studies. Through these pages we can see the evolution of the author's thinking and practice in relational psychotherapy as she explores the multiplicity of selves in the therapeutic engagement, describing a 'way of knowing the other (which) allows for the uniqueness of both in the encounter because it is not fixed, static, or even consistent.'"

Charlotte Sills, *Professor, Integrative Psychotherapist, Teaching and Supervising Transactional Analyst, Coach and Supervisor*

"I had a visceral experience reading Helena's book. I felt in my heart space an expansion and a warm stirring as I accompanied her on her journey. This book, skillfully and successfully demonstrates how the integration of the brain's right and left hemisphere is more than an analytical tool, but one that holds the essence of our creative self, our personalities and our experiences. It therefore succeeds in highlighting the significance of bringing the 'whole self' into relationships.' As I read it, I felt that Helena was giving the gift of her full self to the reader and what a generous gift!"

Hazel Hyslop, *Systemic Psychotherapist, Supervisor, Tutor and Leadership Coach*

"Helena Hargaden has been at the forefront of developing relationality in transactional analysis for many years, about which this volume provides a living testament to the depth of her thinking. This selection, which encompasses a range of subjects, including transgenerational trauma, gender, anniversaries, culture, the relational third, boundaries, endings, money, the erotic, and politics, shows how Hargaden moves seamlessly from the clinical, through reflection, to the imaginative, and the theoretical. In this, we see Hargaden's profound commitment to her clinical work, as well as her creativity in advancing relational theory. The book is lyrical, moving, humorous, and profound, and well deserves its place in this World Library series."

Keith Tudor, *Professor of Psychotherapy, Auckland University of Technology*

"Reading her new book, Helena Hargaden encouraged me to take the road less travelled when it comes to my working and personal life. She makes a strong plea that as Relational Transactional Analysts, apart from using our theoretical knowledge as our main source, we dare to dive into the endless resources of metaphors, literature, music and other creativity housing in the right hemisphere of our brain. It is a joy to read how she actually manages to give clear words to experiences that go beyond words. For me it was like arriving at a tantalizing resting place on my travels."

Mirjam te Slaa, *Transactional Analyst Counseling and Team Coach, BSc Speech therapy, PTSTA-C, The Netherlands*

"This profound, moving book is a must for all psychotherapy training course syllabuses. Not only a fascinating memoir documenting a 30-year career and a journey towards becoming a significant contributor to the workings and theory of relational psychotherapy, particularly in Transactional Analysis, it will also act as a guide for students, qualified psychotherapists and those outside the clinical field. Dr Hargaden's authority, energy, and humility will inspire the reader to use their whole minds, helping them synthesise the non-linear right-hemisphere 'noise' of their subjectivities with their left hemisphere 'theoretical formulations' to bring deeper meaning and understanding into the therapeutic endeavour."

Patrick Brook, *Co-Founder and Academic Director, The Connexus Institute, Hove*

"As in a compilation album, this exciting book offers an enticing collection of the fifteen best hits produced by clinical master Helena Hargaden on both the art and the heart of psychotherapy. The result is an intimate invitation for psychotherapists and clinicians in general to tune the left hemisphere to the right as they read through, and at the same time listen to, a deeply inspiring and moving story of Hargaden's most personal, clinical, academic and creative experience."

Zefiro Mellacqua, *Consultant Psychiatrist and Certified Transactional Analyst (CTA-P), Head of Home Treatment Team, Ticino, Switzerland*

Beyond Language in Relational Psychotherapy

This collection of chapters by Dr. Helena Hargaden makes the case for the evolution of relational theory from a scientific and poetic knowledge base, expressing the different forms of human suffering.

Journal articles, book chapters, and speeches spanning the course of 22 years trace the evolution of the author's own mind alongside the evolution of relational theory. Drawing on her knowledge of science and poetry, Dr. Hargaden examines case studies tracing the relational process, which involves the vulnerability of both therapist and client as change happens in them through complex relatedness. The author makes broad in-depth theoretical links with humanistic and psychoanalytic perspectives, which reveal the richness inherent in the term "Relational." Themes explored include intersubjectivity, the use of the analyst's subjectivity, mutuality, therapy as a two-way street, dissociation, enactment, the use of "the third," race, gender, and sexuality.

Blending approachable language and themes with highly intellectual ideas, this text will be of high value and intrigue to a wide range of readers, particularly transactional analysts and relational psychotherapists.

Helena Hargaden, MSc, D.Psych, TSTA, works and lives in Sussex. She is coeditor and author of a variety of papers and books. She has been widely published and translated into a number of languages. She was awarded the Eric Berne Memorial Award in 2007 for her work with Charlotte Sills on the "domains of transference."

The World Library of Mental Health

The *World Library of Mental Health* celebrates the important contributions to mental health made by leading experts in their individual fields. Each author has compiled a career-long collection of what they consider to be their finest pieces: extracts from books, journals, articles, major theoretical and practical contributions, and salient research findings.

For the first time ever the work of each contributor is presented in a single volume so readers can follow the themes and progress of their work and identify the contributions made to, and the development of, the fields themselves.

Each book in the series features a specially written introduction by the contributor giving an overview of their career, contextualizing their selection within the development of the field, and showing how their own thinking developed over time.

Recent titles in this series:

A Developmentalist's Approach to Research, Theory, and Therapy: The Selected Works of Joseph Lichtenberg
By Joseph D. Lichtenberg

Living Archetypes: The Selected Works of Anthony Stevens
By Anthony Stevens

Soul: Treatment and Recovery: The Selected Works of Murray Stein
By Murray Stein

Existential Psychotherapy and Counselling after Postmodernism: The selected works of Del Loewenthal
By Del Loewenthal

Love the Wild Swan: The Selected Works of Judith Edwards
By Judith Edwards

Beyond Language in Relational Psychotherapy: The Selected Works of Helena Hargaden
By Helena Hargaden

Beyond Language in Relational Psychotherapy

The Selected Works of
Helena Hargaden

Helena Hargaden

Routledge
Taylor & Francis Group

LONDON AND NEW YORK

First published 2023
by Routledge
4 Park Square, Milton Park, Abingdon, Oxon OX14 4RN

and by Routledge
605 Third Avenue, New York, NY 10158

Routledge is an imprint of the Taylor & Francis Group, an informa business

British Library Cataloguing-in-Publication Data
A catalogue record for this book is available from the British Library

ISBN: 978-1-032-26621-3 (hbk)
ISBN: 978-1-032-26622-0 (pbk)
ISBN: 978-1-032-26623-7 (ebk)

DOI: 10.4324/9781032266237

Typeset in Times New Roman
by MPS Limited, Dehradun

For David Freeman

Contents

Acknowledgments

I would never have written this book without Keith Tudor's encouragement and support. Throughout the journey of writing this book, he has companioned and nourished me making it possible for me to stay the course! Thank you to Grace McDonnell from Routledge who has taken me through the tortuous journey of preparing a manuscript ready for publishing. Without her, I could not have prepared this manuscript! Thank you to Shoba Nayar who so generously edited some of my work. Robin Fryer came to my rescue when preparing the manuscript. Just when I was thinking I might have to give up on this project, Robin produced the original articles so I did not need to convert them into Word—a process that was not going well! There would be no book without her help. Thank you so much too to Susan Lockwood who sorted out the required conversion of my diagrams and article, which was refusing to be converted into a readable version of Word.

Gratitude towards the group of qualified psychotherapists and consultants, who joined a study group to discuss six of my articles from the perspective of literature and neuroscience over a period of six month. I appreciated your wholeheartedness especially when it came to making poetic links with the narratives. So thank you to: Gary Bishop, Daniella budisa ubovic, Jane Kiblewhite, Kate Knight-Sands, Rona Rowe, Kareen Ryden, Anthea Snow, Simeon Vellani, Anita Webster, and Elie Williams. Having ascertained that the use of metaphorical language lights up the right hemisphere (Davies, Liverpool University, 2010), we examined the meaning making that cannot happen with just rational thought. We had many of those lightbulb moments!

Thank you to all my colleagues who, over the years, have nourished me through dialogue and connectedness. A very special thank you here to Charlotte Sills. An extremely gifted editor, she generously read my final copy. I am reminded yet again of what feels to be the gift of our collaboration over so many years on so many levels. Thank you to my supervisees, trainees, but most of all to my clients who have provided me with the opportunity to find so much satisfaction and enrich my mind as I continue to evolve.

How many people does it take to write a book? It turns out, quite a lot.

Introduction—Poetry and Metaphor, Literature, and Laughter in Relational Psychotherapy

In this book, I take the opportunity to reflect on 15 articles and talks I have written and presented between 1999 and 2019. The majority of the pieces are case studies, in which I offer personal reflections and autobiographical details that have direct relation to the case.

My reflective writing is connected to the intersubjective, countertransferential relational theories I apply to my work. Inspired by neuroscience, music and literature I explore the world of the non-verbal and non-cognitive ways of experience that bring deeper meaning to the therapeutic relationship. By presenting my work in this manner, I intend to pique the reader's interest in looking for these themes in their own practice and theoretical understanding.

My goal is to recognise how it is our intuitive, creative, and distinctive ways of being in the relational field, which are the source of theoretical and clinical depth and not the other way round. Some of the articles are cow-ritten. In this profession of psychotherapy, every thing we do is collaborative in one way or another. My work with my analyst, colleagues, clients, supervisors, supervisees, and students is an essential part of the mutuality that is the basis of relational theory. I have learned so much from my participation as a writer, psychotherapist, and teacher that I wanted to share some of that collaboration in this book, so I have included some of my published articles, talks and co-authored relational articles where our dialogue is either explicit or implicit.

I begin this introduction by describing the experience of a study group that looked at 6 of the 15 articles in this book from the perspective of each group member. I follow this up with a series of headings in the form of questions based on our group discussions, my personal associations with literature, and my understanding of the connections between the right and left hemispheres of the brain (Damasio, Schore, Stern, McGilchrist). I have used McGilchrist's concept of the divided brain as a way of reflecting on how our minds work. Throughout the introduction, I establish links between the various themes of the chapters set out in this book.

DOI: 10.4324/9781032266237-1

The Study Group

As part of my preparation for this book, I offered to do a short course for the International Association of Relational Transactional Analysis (IARTA). The course was attended by ten qualified psychotherapists who were interested in having a conversation about the links between neuroscience, literature, and my articles and talks. I introduced the group to neuroscientists such as Schore, Damasio, and McGilchrist who variously describe the process of right brain-right brain connection. In McGilchrist's book (2019) *"The Master and His Emissary,"* he describes the brain as divided—with the left hemisphere a more linear source of knowledge and the right hemisphere a source of metaphorical knowledge. In many ways of course the right and left hemispheres are often synthesised as we will understand from the following discussion and collected chapters.

With this understanding as the basis for our group discussions, we initially looked at our work from the perspective of the right hemisphere, making links with poetry, art, and musical lyrics, and then synthesised this knowledge with multiple theoretical connections sometimes associated with a more linear way of thinking. Through our conversations, we began to realise that some theoretical perspectives reflected a synthesis of both left and right hemispheres. Perhaps these theoretical perspectives are the most sympathetic and offer the most valuable contributions to our work as psychotherapists? Throughout this book I invite you, the reader, to make a distinction between those theories you are familiar with which offer this type of synthesis and those that keep strictly to a linear frame of understanding.

Each month, the group would read one of my articles or talks. Together, we made links between the content, the poetry, and lyrics that came to mind in response to reading the article with some added reflections on neuroscientific links which seemed significant. The group responded positively to this process as a starting point, going on to make their own personal and professional connections. I was inspired by their readiness and willingness to express themselves so openly when sharing their poets and lyricists of choice. The following are some of the group discussions we had, as well as my reflections both during and after those discussions.

Upon reading the articles, participants made their own personal connections with poets and music from a wide variety of traditions, including rock music through to poetry, from the Beatles, Elbow, Dylan, Walter de la Mare, Shakespeare, Milton, and many others. As we reflected on the meanings conveyed by poetry and musical lyrics, we realised that metaphor not only catches the essence of the client's nonverbal communication but also frequently eclipses theoretical formulation. The term "unconscious intersubjective relatedness" provides a meta understanding of how metaphor works in our minds. Because unconscious material is held to be co-constructed rather than revealed, the analyst's role is not to avoid personal participation in the process, rather to continually monitor and use the immediate and residual effects of their personal participation as a part of their internal dialectical experience which is not to be shared, but to be reflected on and then maybe translated into a meaingful response.

Our conversations led us to consider the role of musicality in the therapeutic relationship. We came to the conclusion that it is not so much *what* we say as it is *how* we say it that communicates an understanding of the client's mental condition. In this way, the personal is professional. With this in mind, we realised that we will inevitably run into potholes that will lead us into unfamiliar territory and, more often than not, result in a reciprocal acknowledgement of one another's subjectivities, even if only for a little while. Nevertheless, theory forms part of the therapeutic sandwich—we have to synthesise both hemispheres of the brain. One member of the group understood this as his struggle in his therapy to individuate from the negative patriarchal upbringing he had endured, which left him reluctant to think theoretically. He recognised this was something for him to work through and was able to acknowledge how his attitude was hampering his work and that theory was a necessary servant in support of his intuitive mind. It is therefore important to draw on multiple theoretical sources to expand our reflective minds. For instance, in "An Analysis of Nonverbal Transactions Drawing on Theories of Intersubjectivity" (Chapter One), my colleague, Brian Fenton, brought a theoretical perspective of intersubjectivity, which, although different than mine, chimed with my experience, thereby lending richness to our understanding of the case study in the article.

Whilst theory is, of course, vital, we have to be careful not to be dominated by our theoretical understanding. Straying from theoretical certainty can invoke a sense of shame, confusion, and anxiety. For instance, when discussing "The Role of the Imagination in an Analysis of Unconscious Relatedness" (Chapter Two), in which I show how my reverie guides the therapeutic process in a most uncanny way, a member of the group asked "But how can you trust this reverie?" Allowing our imagination into the therapeutic process feels risky as we move into an improvisational mode, inducing a feeling of being "out of bounds," and that such meandering is too private and not relevant. McGilchrist understands this as the Cartesian split, whereby, during the Enlightenment, the inner world was separated from the external world. Stern (1985) views this as separation between non-verbal experience and verbal perceptions of self. In his theory of domains of self, Stern describes the verbal sense of self as typically more concrete and objective, arguing that the verbal sense of self supports a belief system that we can make sense of and "understand everything."

Working with our imagination, however, may necessitate a more disciplined approach to our work where we must find the therapeutic language to support the integrity of our experience. An example of the type of disorientation that can be caused between the therapist's experience of non-verbal communication and the pull towards verbalisation is in "'Father Where Art Thou?' The Significance of Transgenerational Trauma in a Therapy with Luke" (Chapter Three). When feeling oneself to be at sea, it is important for the therapist to feel supported by a fluid theoretical perspective such as Bromberg's (1998) metaphor of "Standing in the Spaces Between Our Different Self-States." This is a non dogmatic creative way to think about varied verbal and non-verbal responses for the therapist to consider.

It was Stern's underlying principles of the domains of self that influenced the chapter "Deconfusion of the Child Ego State: A Relational Perspective" (Hargaden & Sills, 2001; Chapter Four). The book *Transactional Analysis: A Relational Perspective* (2002) was inspired by this chapter, in which we offer a transferential paradigm that allows the therapist to see their responses to their client as valid, deserving of contemplation, and requiring translation in a way that reflects the client's inner reality. Our goal as psychotherapists is to heal this Cartesian division (though we would not have called it that then) and bring about a synthesis of the poetic, metaphorical, melodic, non-linear with facts, information, and theoretical links. We need the freedom to make random connections that do not seem immediately relevant knowing that we can later make connection with theory.

Annie Rogers (2008) refers to Lacanian theory, which she draws on to help her think imaginatively by looking for the *code* behind the language of the client's words. She examines the etymology of words to uncover hidden meanings that are not conscious to the client. The case studies she presents beautifully demonstrate how this disentangling of the meaning shows that "what it seems to be about—is not what it is about." Our group discussions also focused on the relevance of child developmental theories. We now know that optimal attachment experiences facilitate the development of the "emotional" right brain, the core of the self, and thereby emotional wellbeing in later stages of life. The co-creation of a secure attachment regulates the experience of the child. From this experience the child learns to self-regulate their own state.

From the beginning, the baby is relating to the social environment, seeking emotional experience through facial nonverbal communication as demonstrated so vividly by Tronick's (1998) videos on the still face experiments. He shows how an emotional abandonment leads to the deepest sense of frustration, anger, and eventually despair. To develop our subjective phenomenological mind we need another mind to be engaged with our subjective experience. The therapist cannot work relationally if their mind has a rigid attitude to theory, is in denial, or afraid of their own subjectivity, or has not examined their own mind.

A supervisee revealed how he imagined his therapist reading from "page 99" of a theoretical book because there was a lack of any form of feeling or emotion or personal involvement in their words. This is often the case with a type of learned empathic response such as "you sound as if," and "it seems as if"; but this type of clichéd phrase misses the deeper feeling in the room, feeling which might more accurately and relationally be expressed by: "You don't want to talk to me today?" "You are punching me on the nose again!" "You are crying inside-I can feel it." "You wish you could cut my head off with that imaginary sword you are swinging by your side!" "You want me to stay, you want me to go-what am I supposed to do?" "I don't mind you punching me on the nose, but you know, I will give as much as I get." "Okay, so you know more than I do about this-I am searching in the dark." "I know that feeling-it hurts!" Being open to our feelings in these ways takes courage and is the only thing that can truly change the therapeutic direction. In "Come On You Blues! Our Fathers" (Chapter Five), I was awakened out of my comfortable theoretical zone into the depths of a feeling I had not really understood about myself. Only when I was willing to reach into myself could I help my client.

Of course, the learning we have from child development must coexist with the reality of the adult in front of us. Conceptualising the mind as a complex dialectical group of self-states (Bromberg 1998) avoids the infantilisation so prominent in some therapies. In transactional analysis, for example, the Child ego state can sometimes take centre stage as though it is not interconnected to the Adult, or that the Adult ego state can somehow not have the power to engage with its own Child. Relational theory has sometimes been confused with only listening to the Child ego state but that way of thinking is very simplistic. In a way, it boils down to our psychic energy. We can all recognise how an enraged self-state can dominate us and seek to blot out all other self-states. Consciousness enables us to recognise this process, just like a conductor of an orchestra seeks to tune in to each player to bring about a synthesis of musicality. Psychotherapy aims to bring about large parts of the brain that have not been activated to make consciousness more complex and, therefore, more satisfying. Some questions we can ask ourselves include: "Am I a major or am I minor today?" "What am I tuning in to with this client, with myself?" "What music are we making today?" "Why is the client only playing one note?" "What am I supposed to be hearing here?" "How can we incorporate the whole of the orchestra?" "What does this discordant note connecting within me represent?" "How neurodiverse can I be as a therapist?" A client might say, "I don't want to be here today." How do we hear this? Can we allow a discordant note to right itself? "I am glad I came today." Can we listen to "Both sides now" by Joni Mitchell? Can we sit alongside "The Changes" by Bowie?

The aforementioned thoughts capture the essence of my many reflections over the months I worked with the group. The willing participation of group members enabled me to sustain a deep relational connection with my work. Together we all benefited from the rich conversations that emerged by linking the case studies to poetry and science. Throughout our discussions, it became clear that, even so, our starting point had to be ourselves.

"Poetry lies in the meeting of poem and reader, not in the lines and symbols printed on pages of a book. What is essential is ... the thrill, the almost physical emotion that comes with each reading" (Heaney (quoting Borges) 1995, p. 8). Starting with a personal example that comes to me when I read Heaney's remarks, I recollect reading "Easter 1916" by Yeats for my first tutorial when I returned to higher education at the age of 24, in which he conveyed his feelings about the Irish Uprising. I had a visceral emotional reaction to this poetry. Yeats communicated such a range of emotions about the 1916 Uprising while also capturing so much of the situation's ambiguity. As the daughter of an Irish immigrant, I felt proud, anxious, angry, sad, indignant, and outraged. I had not known these feelings until I read this poem. I felt connected to my Irish ancestors and to the beginning of my enquiry into transgenerational trauma.

Who, Am I?

> This above all—to thine own self be true,
> And it must follow, as the night the day,
> Thou canst not then be false to any man.
> (Polonius, in "Hamlet" Shakespeare, 1599–1601)

Who am I exactly? Being and becoming a psychotherapist is built on this foundation. This is a question for which there is no conclusive answer. For instance, I could tell you some facts about myself, such as: I am a woman. Since 1992, I have been a qualified psychotherapist. I began my training at Metanoia (psychotherapy training institute), where I was trained by Petrūska Clarkson, among others. (I relate a ghostly echo of Petrūska that occurred many years after her death when I went to teach at Metanoia Institute in "The Anniversary of the Wailing Woman" (Chapter Six). I was a teacher before that, and my first degree was in English literature. Although I was born in London, I have an Irish passport. I could go on about my personal life, but none of these things will help you get to know me as a person. They might even reinforce prejudice or the notion that you know, understand, and make sense of me. But you would be wrong. Of course, it would provide context for me, but when Bion (1980) taught us to wipe all memory of what we "know" about our client before each session in order to meet each new client anew, he was acknowledging that we find each other through our experiences with the other. Bion was challenging us to see, feel, and know the human person in front of us, and to approach the challenge of meeting an "other from our own point of receptivity and openness. To know someone this way involves having an experience with the person; allowing yourself to have an encounter with the therapist or with the client, that sparks some feelings in both of you. Such an encounter involves the two way street of finding – and maybe even bumping in to – each other to co-create a third or many thirds. This way of knowing the other allows for the uniqueness of both in the encounter because it is not fixed, static, or even consistent. From this perspective, there are two distinct ways of knowing each other. As psychotherapists, it is this second way of knowing that makes us most curious.

What Is This Second Way of Knowing?

To put more flesh on this second way of knowing, we can learn from neuroscience and literature. In 2010, Professor Philip Davis and his team at the Centre for Research into Reading, Information and Linguistic Systems at the University of Liverpool used brain scans to demonstrate that challenging literature 'shifts mental pathways' and prompts new thoughts in readers. Working with the university's magnetic resonance centre, the researchers used scanners to monitor the brain activity of volunteers as they read works by writers such as Shakespeare, Wordsworth, and Eliot. They then "translated" the text into more straightforward, modern language and repeated the test. The scans showed that the original "challenging" literature created much greater electrical activity in the brain, as well as interconnections. Research shows the power of literature to shift mental pathways and create new thoughts, shapes, and connections (McGilchrist 2019).

Poetry is not just a matter of style. It is a matter of deep versions of experience that add the emotional and biographical to the cognitive. This is the argument for serious language in serious literature for serious human situations, instead of self-help books or easy reads that merely reinforce predictable opinions. In Chapter Seven "Anna Karenina, Lilly, and the Cocreated Unconscious Relational Third," I recall a psychotherapy session with a young woman in which none of my theories, including my diagnosis of her narcissism, helped me to connect with her until the fateful day she walked up my street, causing a commotion while reading *Anna Karenina* by Leo Tolstoy. My irritation with her lack of attention to her environment began a prolonged period of disruption in the therapy. By the time we got to the break for summer, I had run out of anything significant to say. I decided to read 'her' book during the summer break. When reading the story of Anna Karenina, I felt as though I was being let in to her inner world. Tolstoy's depiction of Anna's psychological complexity made me feel more curious about my client. There was clearly more to her than she was letting on. My curiosity helped turn the therapy around to travel in a direction that led her into the fertile plains of her own life. The book had provided us both with a metaphor, with the "third," which helped us to move out of the impasse.

McGilchrist (2019) argues that we have learned to dismiss metaphorical knowledge in favour of the left hemisphere, which deals with facts, information, and certainty, despite the fact that the right hemisphere is more prominent in our experience of ourselves. The right hemisphere grows from fetal development to toddlerhood in the first thousand days. From the shape of the brain, we know that there is a developmental need for social experience to bring about psychobiological development, that social connection affects genes, which is now understood as the theory of epi genetics. Imaging shows how the mother's right hemisphere is directly connected to the foetus through the placenta. In compelling language and scholarly erudition, McGilchrist argues that the right hemisphere of the brain is the master and the left hemisphere of the brain is an important servant to the right hemisphere. This has huge implications for culture, education, work, governments, and for our purposes here—psychology and, specifically, psychotherapy. Indeed, the new knowledge that has emerged from neuroscience contributes to the emergence of a paradigm shift in psychotherapy away from cognition and towards emotional relatedness. The research shows how the right hemisphere is more advanced than the left, with 40,000 new synapses developing every second, and this growth is essential to everything else that follows in the brain. The emotional right hemisphere is the core of the self.

Daniel Stern was one of the forerunners of how to think about the evolving brain and where to locate it in relation to our work as psychotherapists. When he published his book *The Interpersonal World of the Infant* (Stern, 1985), he drew on 30 years of collaboration and research into the developing mind. He gave a detailed account of the inner workings of the brain in which he outlined four domains of self; three of which are nonverbal. This way of thinking is supported by other colleagues in our profession. For instance, Ogden (1991, p. 16) wrote "an analytic experience—like all other experiences, does not come to us in words. An analytic experience cannot be told or written; an experience is what it is."

Stern argued that the verbal self often alienates us from the emergent self. Kristeva (1988), a philosopher and psychoanalyst, describes this earliest sense of self as the semiotic. She refers to Lacan's theory that the use of language signifies "the father" who interrupts the symbiosis between mother and child as discussed in Hargaden (2019). Her "semiotic" predated the advances in neuroscience and captures beautifully the nuanced relatedness that involves multi-modal communication including facial expression, intonations, and gestures. These ways of communicating involve emotional relatedness that is more ambiguous and complex than language can be. Meaning is made through perception, sensation, and feelings, forming the basis of our subjectivity. The infant is seeking emotional experience from the very beginning—it is wired into the genome. Tronick's (1998) experiments called "still life" clearly demonstrate this (see further). This is why metaphor conveys so much more than prose ever could.

Are Metaphors an Essential Part of Psychotherapy?

Etymologically, the term "metaphor" derives from the Greek words meta + phenrei meaning "bear, carry" (Charteris-Black 2004, p. 19). From my research into linguistics, it would seem that our language is more redolent of metaphors than we realise; suggesting a type of synthesis between right and left hemispheres whereby language has already evolved to draw attention simultaneously to both facts and our feelings and imaginations. For instance, linguists Knowles and Moon (2006) suggest that idioms and compounds words have metaphorical meanings such as "computer-virus," "miss the boat" and "pigeon-hole." According to Knowles and Moon metaphors can be divided into two types. One type is conventional and used to explain phenomenon so is hand in hand with both our right and left hemispheres. The other type they describe as creative metaphors designed to bring about feelings and suggest something new that cannot be explained. "The essence of creative metaphor is understanding and experiencing one kind of thing in terms of another" (Lakoff & Johnson 1980, p. 5). In psychotherapy, it is the creative metaphor in which we are most interested. This is because analogies capture people's individuality. Metaphors represent the distinctive intersubjectivity of the client-therapist relationship. We discover something new in each other and in our relatedness on this two-way street of connection. We discover meanings that were previously unknown, unidentified, or unnamed. They represent the incomprehensible, the non-verbal, and the unknown. As a result, metaphorical, melodic, non-linear language has evolved into a serious and knowledgeable means of communicating in order to effect psychological shifts and change.

How to Recognise Metaphors in Action

In "Remember, Remember, the Fifth of November" (Chapter Eight), the activity of Guy Fawkes Night created a metaphor through which we were able to conduct the therapy. My client did not know that I too hated Guy Fawkes Night, which originated from the Gunpowder Plot of 1605, a failed conspiracy by a group of provincial English Catholics to assassinate the Protestant King James I of England and VI of Scotland and replace him with a Catholic head of state. I felt her sense of threat, which in her case was from the Nazis, as though it was my own. My expereince of Bonfire Night as it is collouially known in the UK is one of unaccountable depression maybe linked to an unconscious association as a person with Catholic ancestors and my own childhood experience of being attacked because of my religion. Once a year the skies were filled with fireworks, loud noises, flashes of fire, and every year, for five years, we were off into the misty, cloudy, threatening, terrifying world of my client's childhood.

When I first went to my Jungian analyst, who was also a Rabbi, I informed him that I wanted to reconnect with my child who had been raised in Ireland from the ages of two to six. I had no idea I would make this request, but something about his demeanour, his manner of listening, made me feel like this was exactly what I needed to do. He had, it turned out, spent his childhood in Ireland. He had built collegial links with the Christian Brothers in Blackrock College, which was in the neighbourhood where I had lived as a child. This was a synchronous experience. A synchronous experience is understood as the simultaneous occurrence of events that appear significantly related but have no discernible causal connection. When he referred to his experience in Ireland, I felt known in some way. He knew the cultural lexicon; he had been steeped in it and then intellectually engaged with the religiosity of the Irish people, just as I had. I had lived with a great aunt who had been a head school teacher. I had an experience of a religious and intellectual mind. My analyst used language in a way I felt as rhythmic or musical. It transpired that he was a musician (so am I). In this way, I had the experience of being met and received before actually knowing it more consciously as a fact. His way of listening offered a poetic, more musical space rather than an analytic one.

Kristever (1969/1980) associates the poetic with the maternal body. During this time, I recall feeling him so deeply in my body and in my heart, especially when I was curled up in a fetal position at night before going to sleep. None of these experiences were explicitly spoken about. I knew that it was related to my earliest trauma, which was my abandonment as a baby. This was sadly linked to an experience I had, which was no one's fault or intention. It was one of those accidents that caused psychological damage when my mother and I were separated for a month when both of us were hospitalised for different illnesses. I came to know about it through my mother telling me how, when she came to collect me from the hospital after a month's separation, I did not know her. I had lost her and could not reconnect with her. I used to feel sorry for my mother; now I know how this deepest of wounds played out in my life quite unconsciously and, as I say, with no one to blame. Soon after beginning psychotherapy, I had a dream in which I travelled in a boat to the other side of the world. This was clearly a symbol for the type of journey I had embarked upon with my analyst, taking me away from causality, information, facts, and mechanisms and into the unknown forest of images and feelings. In this way, I became involved in an intuitive and imaginative process with my analyst who was a linguist, religious, imaginative, and yet rooted in a deep sense of his own consciousness.

During this analysis, my mind was reshaped by the types of poetic multimodal meanderings referred to by Kristever. The journey enabled me to develop a confidence in my intuitive critiques of conceptual ideas and theoretical models. It was this evolutionary process that lead to collaborating with my colleague Charlotte Sills and the publication of our book *Transactional*

Analysis: A Relational Perspective (Hargaden & Sills, 2002) in which we proposed a different type of conversation about the nature of relatedness from the transactional view, which was rooted in cognitive behavioural change. In our theoretical formation of the domains of transference we suggested that change can only occur through a transferential process. We set out to demonstrate how the two subjectivities of both therapist and client are implicated in bringing about lasting change in the mind of the client and the therapist. Nothing changes if the therapist does not change. Unsurprisingly, our relational model influenced many collegial conversations and critiques. Overall, our community showed how much they both resonated with and valued our relational ideas by giving us the Eric Berne Memorial Award in 2005. Of course no "man" or therapeutic modality is an island to him/itself and, as it turned out, other modalities were having similar types of conversations. We were part of the zeitgeist.

There was a sense of synchronicity and mutuality in the way our thinking was reflected in other modalities. Other colleagues from different modalities were turning to their theoretical models and challenging the received wisdom that psychological change happens through disembodied interpretations or by sharing and explaining conceptual understanding, or even by learning how to respond empathically as though this could be learned. For instance, McGilchrist argues that the left hemisphere can demonstrate empathy but it is more superficial in contrast with the right hemisphere which is more in touch with primary-process emotionality. In "Building Resilience: The Role of Firm Boundaries and the Third in Relational Group Therapy" (Chapter Nine), I make a distinction between the more learnt empathic responding and the more primitive process of attunement. Guggenbuhl Craig (1971) describes empathy as a potentially potent mechanism for taking control and manipulating others. Unfortunately, empathy is often taught as a technique. When used in this way, it gives the very false idea that the therapist actually understands the client. This process is not necessarily happening at all but does make the therapist appear powerful and in control. A supervisee who had trained in several establishments and gained a counselling qualification recently described how his former therapist rolled out what he thought of as clichés because his felt experience was there was no emotionality in the interaction. According to McGilchrist, the left hemisphere is primarily concerned with power and is over confident in its own sense of what is reality. The misuse of empathy in this way suggests the shadow side of our profession.

How Subjectivity Is Formed in the Right Hemisphere of the Brain

Beebe (2002), Harrison (2011, 2014), Seligman (2017), Tronick (2007), and others chart and examine the developing and evolving brain that forms the basis of our subjectivity. Infant research shows that the quality of interactions form and build one's identity/sense of self, detailing the complex process of self-regulation and dyadic regulation of emotions, intentions, and behaviours. According to McGilchrist (1991), early development is the basis of the right hemisphere of the brain, which is larger than the left hemisphere. The relational alliance does not go through the neocortex (Schore, 2012). It is clear that the nature of the therapist, who they are as a person, their ethical values, and the extent of their self examination, will communicate itself unconsciously to the client. It turns out that relationship is a two-way street. Who would have thought it? The poets knew this and have communicated their feelings about the mysteries of being human through poetry since time immemorial.

Transformational Transference (Hargaden & Sills, 2002)

Melanie Klein's (1946) theory of projective identification attempts to bring us into the internal experiences of the infant, of the right hemisphere. Her theories of good and bad breast, splitting, and envy offered ways of thinking about the internal mind of the infant before we had corroboration from science. However, the way this theory is used tends to objectify the therapist as someone who can get the meaning of the projective identification without feeling it; a conceptual theory by which the therapist can remain hidden, even from themselves. The therapist is apparently meant to respond with a disembodied interpretation that makes it clear that what the client is projecting into the therapist is nothing to do with the therapist. It is, of course, a self-protective mechanism to keep the therapist as a type of perfect object. Given that the mind evolves through a process of intersubjectivity with another, it is clear that projective identification is a process that has to involve the therapist in the feeling parts of themselves. In the domains of transference, we suggest that the therapist needs to recognise areas of themselves that they find disturbing. In this way, they do not understand their client as much as they "get" their client's experience. This requires a non-defensive but nevertheless thoughtful approach, which we described as the transformational transference.

"When Parting Is Not Such Sweet Sorrow" (Chapter Ten) shows how the projective process can be both deeply moving and profoundly disturbing at the same time. In many ways, the transformational process is a mysterious one best described metaphorically. In the song "Mr Tambourine Man," Bob Dylan invites us to follow the tambourine man on a journey using evocative metaphors that I would encourage you to look up for yourselves as I don't have the copyright to repeat the wonderful imagery he uses in which Dylan captures the madness and poetic truth of the type of journey we begin with our clients if we are willing and able. It involves a move away from certainty yet with a spirit of integrity and willingness to be on the journey. As relational psychotherapists we are required to work with the dialectic clamouring and noise of our self-states. We are called upon to examine our varied self-states, make meaning from them and turn to the servant of our minds, the left hemisphere, for theoretical ballast. This is quite an exacting task in which we are required to synthesise the right and left hemispheres of our brains. We are called upon to draw on the wisdom of the right hemisphere whilst checking in with the left hemisphere. We are required to provide a container which can hold both memory and fate.

How Theory Can Negate the Right Hemisphere of the Brain

In my view, a tragic example of a complete negation of the right hemisphere was enacted by the (UK) National Health Service when it decided to get rid of humanistic, arts, and psychoanalytic psychotherapists and wheel in a band of newly qualified and minimally trained cognitive behavioural therapists. It was argued that troubled people could change their thinking and behaviour—a process which would solve their problems. The evidence for this outrageous decision was not considered at all by the person who inspired these changes. He was able to influence these changes because he was a member of the House of Lords. If any good is done by cognitive behavioural therapists it is through their value as a human being and their innate ability to attune to their clients; not through their theory of change which does not stand up to scientific examination.

The relational approach, however, might be highly upsetting to a therapist who has not been curious enough to persist in a self-examination process. The clues the client picks up about the therapist's state of mind will resonate throughout the therapy, and the therapist will have no control over it. For example, in many of the case studies in this book, I am migrated out of my comfort zone into uncharted country. I am forced to either be open to or guard against other aspects of myself by turning to clichéd theoretical replies.

Can There Be Theory Without Love: Can There be Love Without Theory

Theory gives us a place to return as we navigate through the forests of our minds, where sorrows and disturbing experiences within ourselves and our clients reveal themselves in crazy patterns of feelings and thoughts. Such a process demands us to explore the vast universe of theoretical knowledge that now exists. We cannot afford to stay married to one theory or way of thinking. The process of drawing on multiple theoretical perspectives mirrors the dialectical nature of the mind whilst at the same time reflecting our contemporaneous understanding of cultural concerns and recent neuroscientific discoveries. In *Transactional Analysis: A Relational Perspective* (Hargaden & Sills, 2002), we focus on the idea of the therapist's subjectivity as the initial phase of beginning to "find our client in ourselves" (Bollas, 2000, p. 202). This means to use our heart, our attunement, to draw on our own history of trauma and to convert it, translate it, make meaningful connection with the client. Thomas Szasz (1960) maintains that unlike true disease of the brain and body, mental illness is a destructive social construct that medicalises living and deprives people of their dignity. According to Szasz, medication, hospitalisation, and mandated psychotherapy are little more than coercive, dignity-reducing forms of clinical practice with an emphasis upon diagnosis. While this method of thinking has certain merits, it appears to me to guarantee the superiority of the therapist's "knowledge" without them having any evident ownership of their own disturbed self states.

An over reliance on pathology creates a distance by placing the damage a step away from ourselves. However, if we take, as a starting point, the therapist's knowledge of their own complex dialectical world, we can assume they will have a broad and wide relationship with multiple theoretical formulations. For it is through their silent inner processing that they can expand, observe their experience, and, by doing so, offer an implicit invitation to the client to feel invited and welcomed (Kristever 1994). No theory can replace the therapist's intention to work with their client thoughtfully, compassionately, and lovingly. At the same time, such intentionality will not suffice if the therapist is wary of theory. The right hemisphere values genuine, lyrical metaphorical interaction, while the left hemisphere backs it up with data, facts, information, and the ability to synthesise by combining the two forms of knowledge.

In recent years, I have taken from many relational and Jungian psychoanalysts new metaphors that capture the heartfelt journey in which we are engaged. Metaphors such as "airless worlds," "companioning," "feelings matter," "relational unconscious," "surrender," "the developmental third" (other thirds), "the bi directionality of the relational unconscious," "transformation," "Negre to gold," "anima and animus," "the infinity of the unsaid," are only a few examples. When metaphorical language is employed in this way, it captures a wide range of theoretical ideas and language, providing us with a synthesis of both the right and left hemispheres. Many of these writings are beautifully expressed, and while they do not necessarily say anything new, they frequently integrate heart, soul, and the rigour of reflective minds, putting the poetic on centre stage of our work. Metaphors assist us in bridging the gap between talking about and experiencing relatedness.

The Art of Improvisation—What a Difference a Word Makes

Tronick (2007), Beebe (2002), and Stern et al. (1986) researched the mutual regulation of interactions between parent and infant as well as between adults. We now know how dyadic interactions consist of ongoing emotional exchanges of verbal and nonverbal information which enable self-regulation and mutual regulation. Meanings are co-created by therapist and client. A client has a dream of a beautiful house, but they only reside in one room. The house is full of rooms but they do not know them. We have to go off-piste to find out what is in these other rooms of her psyche. This can feel risky; yet involves an essential part of our deepest subjectivity which is often embedded in humour. There is space here for playfulness, for the therapist to risk going into a place they do not know so that the client can also take the risk.

I am reminded of my 16-year-old son who was moaning, groaning, and letting me know that as far as he was concerned I clearly knew nothing, understood nothing, and was a very annoying and irritating "other" in his life. Of course I felt the blow and found myself responding without much thought but straight to the point he was making: "Daniel, it must be very difficult living with a retard." He was about to answer back with a stinging retort when he suddenly got the joke and burst out laughing. We re-connected through humour – the gift of the right hemisphere! With a client, recently, I suggested that they were in their teenage self in response to them disregarding, yet again, something I was saying. They responded by saying that it sounded like I was in my teenage self. This caused us both to laugh and again it broke the binary impasse enabling us to reconnect. I had unconsciously revealed something about myself. Yet, for them to say this to me and bring a connection between us was a joyful and positive moment. We were both speaking the same language; we had to find it—it did not happen through theory but through the mutual regulation of interactions. Later, we made meanings that went deep and purposeful into the heart of their sorrow at being denied, negated, and viciously punished for their smart retorts to their criminal father. At a previous time, and I still do this sometimes, as the aforementioned client pointed out, I resort to theoretical formulations which, as you will see in my article "When Parting Is Not Such Sweet Sorrow" (Chapter Ten) are more or less pointless. Indeed they indicate that the therapist is trying to hide! And I was!

"That Was Our Best Session to Date"—The Isolated Landscape

When I was in my second year as a student of transactional analysis, I had a memorable session with a client in which I learned something that was completely absent from the therapeutic curriculum. In my article "To Be or Not to Be—Is That the Question? The Paradox of Script" (Chapter Eleven), for the transactional analysis Cumbrian Conference in 2015, I describe this experience and still, to this day, decades later, I recall the last words my client said as they left the room, buttoning up their too tight jacket, clutching their briefcase, before bending over me, as I sat in my chair.

Looking me directly in the eye, they said "that was our best session yet." How amazing this felt to me at the time when I had not resorted to any theory, but had been in my abandoned self state because of being awake all night with my sick son. My experience with my son had stopped me in my theoretical tracks. It had triggered my feelings of abandonment as a baby about which I knew nothing at the time. It was this vulnerability, sensitivity, loss, anguish, and emotional pain in me that my client had felt, which matched his non-verbalised experiences of loss. We had unwittingly moved into improvisational mode. I had let go of circles and he let go of Bartok, his favourite musician, through which he had tried to describe his pain, but in such abstract terms I was left none the wiser until this fateful day.

In "A Talk on Money, Race, and the links with Karpman's Triangle" (Chapter Twelve), I find myself wrong footed and totally out of my comfort zone. In "Money," I am transported, by virtue of the client's projection, into a royal personage. He did not consciously know that as a baby, abandoned in hospital, the staff had called me the Queen because I stood at the end of my bed with my nose in the air, sighing. He had come from origins in which his whole culture and race had been enslaved and abandoned. We had something in common. From lowly status, we occupied the highest status. By being able to project such worth onto me he found the king inside of himself. The process was extraordinary and connected us both, strangely, to finding our ordinary selves.

I first learned about improvisation in my young days as a drama student studying the theories of improvisation by the Russian dramatist Konstantin Stanislavski. Improvisation brings us into the 'present moment' (Stern 1986). We move 'out of ourselves' into a new emerging space in which no one can say what will happen next. It provides the space for ruptures and repairs to happen. It relies on the therapist's ability and willingness to forgo their shield of theoretical protection, be open to their vulnerability, and be attuned to, and trusting of, the dialect of their own mind.

In "The Erotic Relational Matrix Revisited" (Chapter Thirteen), I trace the type of ethical container we need to hold, particularly when working in the relational field and in particular when "playing" in the improvisational model. In the following extract, we are both in the improvisational space.

Client Tom:	I had an argument with another cyclist this morning. He swerved deliberately into me. Although I kept my cool I let him know exactly what I thought about him.
Me:	Hmm, how did he take that?
Tom:	He started to argue with me and frankly I could have taken his head off with one swipe.
Me:	Sounds nasty. If that had been a woman how would that have played out.
Tom:	You being sexist?

Me:	Er, yes, possibly, but still hey, seriously what would you have felt then do you think?
Tom:	Well, for fucks sake, that is a typical woman's response – that was my mother to a T – bang in to you and then make it something bad about me. Hmm!!!
Me:	How fucking annoying that can be – passive aggression – I often get caught out by that myself.
Tom:	Yeah, you tend to be direct don't you. I punch you on the nose and you punch me back. (Laughs)
Me:	(Laugh)

We connect through the laughter and get back to what was underneath the utter despair he experienced with his disengaged and passive aggressive mother. I become his mother and not his mother because I enter the fight. Ringstrom (2012) tells us not to be afraid of improvisation. He argues that to tip-toe around traumatised clients is to neglect and not see positive self-states in them that can rise to the occasion during this time; self-states that they discover about themselves that are then validated through the process.

Naturally, working in this way will inevitably allow for ruptures but then we can also have the repair because the therapist is not the original abuser. In my aforementioned example, we found untold grief, loss, and despair and this was also alongside the type of resilience discovered in our 'nose to nose' fight. Of course if we choose the improvisational way, we have to be conscious of our own narcissism and certainly improvisation will take a swipe at us—we will no longer be that "perfect mirror." Instead, we become another human being in the encounter with each other in the search for self. I think improvisation also opens up many choices for other types of interventions that are not explicit but carried through the emotional tone of the exchange such as "that is so fucking annoying." I get it.

So What Now?

Of the 15 articles and talks in this book, 7 detail case histories which, when I delivered them, often made people feel something. For example, in "Come on You Blues! Fathers" (Chapter Five), I had written a piece with an open heart, and integrated the image, and to a certain extent the life, of my father into the case history. As I concluded my talk, I was surprised to see members of the audience with tears in their eyes. In those moments, I felt that my sadness for my father, for my client, was validated in a way that did not require words. As the cases turn into articles, there is more of a synthesis between feelings, reflections, non-linear process, and theoretical formulations.

The process of returning to my work in this way has humbled me. I am reminded of the people I have seen over 30 years in my practice and think that what I mostly offered, when I was able, was *Moments of Meeting* (Stern 1986). I am reminded of my talk "Then We'll Come From the Shadows" (Chapter Fourteen), when I again saw tears in the eyes of a colleague whom I had thought probably could not shed tears! Ever! I felt pleased to have connected with them in this way. Again no words—just feelings.

I end finally with a very different type of article. In (Chapter Fifteen), in 2016, colleague Keith Tudor invited me to co write an article with him to commemorate the Easter Uprising in Ireland of 1916. This offered me the opportunity to express some very different thoughts and ideas that I had not been fully aware of. Thoughts which make a connection between politics and psychology, between Victimhood and authentic suffering, between Persecution and Autonomy. All is revealed in the article.

Upon reflection, I think our profession is grandiose in many ways—speaking, writing, and talking as if we can actually make a difference. Many of us do but it is hard to measure. People come and go, people stay; people tell their stories, many of which are harrowing, making us ask ourselves, how can people behave in these cruel ways? We are faced again and again with the mystery of life, the unknowability of human beings, the uncertainty, the crazy sorrows of existence. What makes us want to do this work as psychotherapists? Many of my colleagues moved on from this way of working often moving into consultancy, coaching, training, or just retiring. Why do I do it? I recall a training course I attended many years ago when the tutor asked this type of question and I replied, without thinking, that I had been doing it since I was two! There is some truth in this. I was in training as the eldest of four children but, as I often quip, as the eldest of six because my parents were young and unlearned. For me, there is also the inherited transgenerational trauma of my Irish background, my mother's family trauma, my father's physical trauma from polio, his lyrical non linear mind, all of which has been the stuff of my 28-year analysis. I basically just love my work. I love thinking, meditating, wondering, using myself, my trauma, my leaning towards literature, drama, stories and I find, or seem to find, I can bring about some transformation. Rereading my talks and articles I can see that in many ways it is all about me trying to work out the mysteries of being. I still have not found the answer! Neither has Eigen (2007)—"I wouldn't be surprised to learn that the human race is chemically unbalanced" (p. 54). I laughed at this statement and saw the truth in it!

In the following articles and talks, I look at each chapter and offer some reflections on what it was that inspired me to write the article. I hope this will spur other psychotherapists, in training, and qualified, to value their mind, examine their mind and to consider sharing their work too.

Chapter 1

An Analysis of Nonverbal Transactions Drawing on Theories of Intersubjectivity

Helena Hargaden and Brian Fenton

Relational psychoanalysis—influenced by the interpersonal writings of Sullivan (1953), Thompson (1956/1964), and Fromm (1960); the self psychology of Kohut (1971); and the feminist interpretations of Chodorow (1978), Benjamin (1988), Goldner (1991), and others—developed in a distinct fashion that moved away from the rigid Freudian psychoanalysis more popular in Eric Berne's day.

Within transactional analysis, we consider that the second-order structural model of ego states provides a developmental model appropriate to such a psychoanalytic and relational perspective. In this model, the transferential relationship is central to the clinical work, as shown by Moiso (1985), Novellino (1990), Hargaden and Sills (2002), and others. In addition, we think that the transactional analysis model of ego states foreshadowed current developments within psychoanalysis in terms of movement toward an intersubjective psychology (e.g., Mitchell, 1988; Stolorow, 1995, etc.). By setting up a transactional situation in which two or more people engage with each other, Berne moved away from a one-person psychology toward a two-person psychology that was inherently interpersonal in style. In his transactional analysis model, the analyst is meant to participate in the psychotherapy; hence Berne's suggestion that therapists ask themselves not "Am I in a game? but "Which game am I in?"

In teaching us to think like this, Berne implicated the subjectivity of the therapist and took us to the heart of the meaning of countertransference. At the moment of asking ourselves that question, we have to think about our feelings, thoughts, and beliefs and what is going on within us. Berne (1966/1994), however, retained a focus on the functional aspects of the therapeutic relationship. He stopped short of a deeper inquiry into the subjectivity of the therapist's experience; for instance, he did not require therapists to explore their past and present subjective experience, which may impact the here-and-now relational experience between client and therapist. Instead, possibly influenced by his Freudian past, Berne emphasized the need for therapists to remain observant using their special powers of observation. He described the clinical qualities required of

DOI: 10.4324/9781032266237-2

therapists with characteristic brevity: "observation, equanimity, and initiative" (p. 65). Thus, psychotherapists participate in the interpersonal situation to the extent that they ask themselves what game they are in, but the subjectivity of the therapist, although one aspect of ego state diagnosis, was not emphasized as such in Berne's writing. Rather, he expected the therapist to find out what is happening with the client and to make incisive interventions.

Without necessarily being conscious of the fact, Berne provided a model in which different theories about and perspectives on the client—both as subject and as object—can coexist. Although he continued to stress the importance of observation with a view to objectivity, in moving from a one-person psychology as in classical Freudian analysis—where the patient lay on a couch and the psychoanalyst made interpretations—Berne's model represents movement toward a multiperson psychology. He set up an interpersonal transactional situation that inherently implies a two-person or multiperson psychology in which the therapist's and client's subjective experiences could be further explored and in which the client and therapist can both be seen as subject and object. There is, therefore, an implicit flexibility in the theoretical model of transactional analysis.

Recently, Stark (1998) elaborated three types of psychological relationship: one person, as in the classical Freudian model; one and a half persons, where there is a more interpersonal participation between therapist and client; and two persons, in which there is an emphasis on the reciprocal, mutual relating process. We think that the transactional analysis model lends itself to all three ways of working, depending on the nature of the client's presentation and intention in psychotherapy.

Over the past two decades, there has been an increasing focus within the transactional analysis literature on the subjectivity of the therapist in terms of what is happening for him or her within the relationship. For instance, we now understand the development of script to be reciprocal and based on mutuality (Cornell, 1988). Developments in neuroscience suggest a dyadic, mutually regulating process by which the sense of self is developed (Allen, 2000). The subjectivity of the therapist has come under increasing clinical scrutiny (Hargaden & Sills, 2002; Novellino, 1990) and has been reconceptualized as a cocreated one (Summers & Tudor, 2000). This evolution of relational transactional analysis over the past 20 years extends transactional analysis toward a two-person or multiperson psychology. The person of the therapist, and the dyadic process between the two subjectivities, has become a central issue when thinking about how to bring about significant psychological and social change.

Drawing on this canon of relational thinking, we seek to show how an understanding of the intersubjective relationship—with a particular emphasis on the nonverbal domain of transactions—is clinically imperative to maximize conditions in which fundamental change can occur. We wish to stress that nonverbal does not necessarily mean silent or nonsymbolic; for instance, gestures and sounds can also create symbolic meaning. Most therapists will recognize the existence of nonverbal phenomenon, such as the making of sucking or gurgling noises, pacing and type of breathing, movement of the body into certain positions (e.g., fetal) or sitting forward or moving backward, the use of eye contact and lack of eye contact, and the opening of the mouth to tell one story while the eyes tell something different. In more extreme cases, there are clients who do not turn up or phone or who turn up late or bring something into the room, such as the smell of alcohol, cigarette smoke, or even dog shit on their shoes!

And what about therapists and their nonverbal behavior? They may find themselves involuntarily sighing, drifting off, moving in the chair, defending their body, changing their breathing, or experiencing their heart beating faster or slower. Maybe they forget an appointment, are late, or cannot remember the client's name.

To examine the intersubjective frame, we must ask questions such as, what is the nature of the interaction between therapist and client? For example, is the adoption of a fetal position by the client a response to a look of tenderness in the therapist's eyes? Is that look of tenderness a response to an unconsciously communicated yearning for nurturing? Is the client's anger with the therapist a response to her looking at the clock? Is the therapist unwittingly looking at the clock because she senses anxiety in the client? A further question is, what happens within the emotional atmosphere co-created by the analytic couple? For instance, what makes up the emotional ether of this couple? Is there a sense of companionship, tension, anxiety, or something else? How does this atmosphere change and what does it mean?

Intersubjectivity

The term "intersubjective" has various meanings. One major distinction is intersubjectivity as a developmental achievement as opposed to intersubjectivity as a relational pattern that emerges between two or more subjectivities. We take the view that both of these meanings are relevant to the clinical relationship. Features of intersubjectivity are as follows:

1   It involves mutuality, meaning that both parties unconsciously influence each other emotionally and psychologically. Beebe, Jaffe, and Lachmann (1992) stress that mutuality is not the same as harmony, synchronicity, or attunement. For example, they observed infant and caretaker to be in mutually affecting relationships that moved in and out of synchronicity, contact, ruptures, and repairs.
2   It is dialectic interplay between conscious and unconscious forms of relatedness, as, for example, a conflict between what is believed and what is felt. Such dynamics involve interplay between contact, connection, ruptures, and interpersonal losses.

3   It happens mostly outside of our conscious awareness and involves both participants in an emotional, psychological, and physiological relational experience in which each person constantly affects the other. A simple example of this is sitting with a client and noticing your own and your client's breathing patterns and how they subtly change as you sit together. This reciprocal influence and mutual regulation underpins the very notion of intersubjective relatedness.

The term "intersubjectivity" originates from a philosophical view of human existence that we briefly discuss further. We then turn our attention to recent research within developmental psychology and finally consider the relevance of this research for the clinical situation, which we think is vital for fundamental change to occur in psychotherapy.

Inherent in the theory of intersubjectivity is the phenomenological philosophical view of human existence, which posits that all experience is subjective experience (Husserl, as cited in Marion, 1998) and questions the idea of the individual as an entity. For Sullivan (1953), the notion of unique individuality is an illusion. This perspective suggests a backdrop of core relatedness as an existential given, which provides a relational foundation for existence and is consistent with the findings of prominent infant researchers.

Developmental Perspectives on

Intersubjectivity

Over the past 30 years, developmental researchers have begun to describe an infant who is infinitely more complex, sophisticated, and proactive than had hitherto been thought. Until Stern (1985) presented his findings from infant observation, the psychotherapeutic view of infancy was mostly obtained through analysis of adult experience. The interpersonal infant provides us with another perspective. Stern, using advanced technology, takes us as far as possible into the heart of the subjective life of the infant. His scholarly depiction of an interpersonal infant indisputably shows us that human beings are engaged in a mutually reciprocal relationship from the beginning of life. The discovery of the interpersonal infant requires us to understand the significance of subjectivity while at the same time implicitly challenging the primacy of objectivity.

A significant figure in the shift toward a multiperson psychology is Vygotsky, a social constructionist and infant researcher. Whereas developmental researchers such as Piaget emphasized the individual and staged nature of development through interaction with the environment, Vygotsky—while recognizing a natural line of development—describes and focuses on an intersubjective realm of relatedness. His research moved away from the self as separate and individual to the idea of the self developing through relationship with another. For Vygotsky (1962), the capacity of the infant to develop an organizing subjective perspective about self and others is dependent on the mother's empathic involvement with her infant. She draws the infant into her world of meanings. For Vygotsky (1988), concepts such as language, voluntary attention, and memory are functions that originate in interaction; "the very mechanism underlying higher mental functions is a copy from social interaction; all higher mental functions are internalised social relationships" (p. 74). For Vygotsky, the mother acts as a funnel for culture, and he is interested foremost in the formative influence of society as mediated by the (m)other.

Vygotsky (1978) describes a "zone of proximal development" (ZPD) (p. 86), which is the difference between what a child could have achieved unaided and what he or she can manage with a competent peer; hence, learning itself, to Vygotsky, is relational. His focus is mainly on verbal interaction, but research has shown that versions of ZPD can be observed in much earlier and preverbal relational dyads. Effective mothering involves a sensitive attunement to the infant's movements, gaze, gestures, and vocalizations, and mothers can be seen to take charge of their infants' learning. For example, Newson and Newson (as cited in Oates, 1994) state that the resulting sequence of the infant is a combination of its own activity and an intelligent manipulation of that activity by the much more sophisticated adult partner. The adult, by being contingently responsive to the infant in a way which only another human being could be, manages to hold the infant's attention and to shape the course of his ongoing activity pattern (p. 284).

Bruner (1981, pp. 48–49) describes mothers who are engaged in this process as providing scaffolding within which the child's abilities can be constructed. Through this process, the infant can start to initiate joint attention to objects by drawing her (the caretaker's) attention to them. For example, by patting the object while holding eye contact, "there is present from a surprisingly early pre-linguistic age a mutual system by which joint selective attention between infant and his caretaker is assured—under the control of the caretaker or of the child" (Bruner, 1977, p. 276).

Vygotsky's work with infants is compatible with recent psychoanalytic contributions by Diamond and Marrone (2003). They suggest the term "cothinking" (p. 125) to describe how thinking itself (i.e., the ability to make meaningful links between ideas and between ideas and affect) and the capacity for reflexive function (which they define as "the individual's capacity to perceive, interpret, and respond to another person's mental state and—following from this—the ability to distinguish inner from outer reality" [p. 125]) develop within the relational matrix. Like Vygotsky, they challenge the notion of a single subjectivity and, in doing so, highlight the shared nature of our seemingly individual minds and selves.

Trevarthen (1979, 1984, 1993), a developmental psychologist and biologist, suggests that intersubjectivity is not learned but exists from the beginning as a human capacity. He proposes that we are born with the innate ability to interact; however, the shaping of these interactional styles is heavily contingent on the infant/carer dyad. He moves away from language as the basis of this interaction to focus more on emotion as the communication mode in the building blocks of both language and the self. Trevarthen and others report that the sharing of affective moods and states comes before the sharing of mental states that refer to objects outside of the dyad.

For Trevarthen, a crucial element of intersubjectivity is the sharing of minds, a process by which information is shared and inferred. This process was implied by Freud in his theory of transference and later described as projective identification (Ogden, 1992); we suggest it is also implicit in Berne's theories of ulterior transactions and games. Trevarthen does not postulate the capacity for logical thought as providing the foundations for language; for him linguistic capacities arise from a prereflective innate state of being in which affective states are expressed in gestures that provide emotional interpersonal understanding. This then is the basis for cocreation and emergence of meaning and the precursor of language itself. Early interactions between mothers and infants have been termed "proto-conversations" (Bateson, as cited in Miell & Dallos, 1996, p. 108), and these, although nonverbal, are regarded as embodying the fundamentals of the verbal conversations of older children and adults.

Primary Intersubjectivity

Trevarthen (1979) categorizes intersubjectivity into two main components, which are primary and secondary intersubjectivity. Primary intersubjectivity (zero to six months) describes a form of presymbolic interaction and a phase of development with the function of the interchanges primarily being the development of sensitivity in the baby to the subjective experience of the (m)other. This is coupled with awareness that the mother can also be sensitive to the subjective experience of the infant. In effect, there is a "meeting of minds."

Development of this ability is contingent on the quality of attuned interaction within the relational context between caretakers and infant. Examples of these interchanges are early proto-conversations, such as mimicry and turn taking. The rhythm of the exchanges is crucial. From this process comes the development of the capacity to share emotional meaning. Affective states are expressed as vocalizations; gesture and the rhythm of the exchange, timing and synchronicity, and musicality are emphasized as these are the sensory means of creating relation and affect. From this attunement, shared meaning emerges (Stern, 1985).

Within this space, there is a third subjectivity that is neither mother nor infant, one in which the infant directly accesses the adult's emotional experience, and the adult senses and contains the infant's emotional states—in other words, a space that is created between infant and caretaker. This dyadic process highlights the notion of a shared mind, meaning a shared subjectivity. We postulate that this pathway is the conduit through which our sense of self is cocreated. By utilizing the early dyadic interchanges discussed earlier (i.e., communication through the senses), we are able to coconstruct meaning of self and other and thus form our primary sense of self, which is literally a "felt" sense. These exchanges continue into adulthood and can be seen to be the basis for transforming our sense of who we are through further immediate here-and-now relational experiences.

Trevarthen (1993) views emotional development as a process to which both parties bring qualities, skills, and expectations:

> Infant communications are better co-ordinated, more regular, more elaborate and more evocative and productive when they are being responded to by a partner who shows positive empathy. This means that the infant is prepared to participate as one actor in a "dialogic" exchange or "closure" of feelings that has a certain quality of richness .... The infant is not merely seeking any kind of contingent events ... or recurrent forms of stimulation of a given physical intensity or richness. (p. 68)

That the infant prefers empathy and seeks out empathic responsiveness is interesting but not surprising. It is worth focusing for a moment on the preferred status of empathic transactions and ponder what this might mean in relation to intersubjective experiences. We suggest that what Trevarthen (1993) means when he goes on to stipulate that we as humans have "special empathic properties" (p. 68) can be directly related to the experience, in the coconstruction of self, of the sharing of mind. For example, if the core self is indeed constructed in part through conscious and unconscious imitations and identifications with the other, then this empathic quality would surely make these experiences possible in the first place, and the more developed one becomes in these types of reflexive abilities, the more able one will be to share the other's mind. This would seem to have the developmental advantage of making self-constructive experiences more likely.

From Trevarthen's work, we see that infant and caretaker are in conversation long before language develops. He suggests that emotions are central ingredients of early relationships, with mother and baby continually reacting and adjusting to each other at an emotional level. However, he postulates that emotions are not simply in the mother or the baby but are essentially a part of the process between them. In other words, we could say that the relationship between two individuals contains more than the sum of the parts.

All human emotions are capable of changing another person's feelings and motives. Whatever its other functions in defending vital processes, or regulating action on the world and cognitive operations inside a subject, including self-awareness, every emotion that is expressed can directly and immediately affect emotions in another person (Trevarthen, 1993, p. 2).

The immediacy and direct effect of the emotional exchanges within the primary intersubjective process is an important idea to grasp. It is not until later in development (see secondary intersubjectivity below) that attention is moved away from the "core sense of self" constructive influences of the immediate relational experience. The aforementioned quote describes a third coconstructed subjectivity, something that exists in the shared space between infant and caretaker, and suggests that we can, therefore, make people feel things and them us. This notion is extended by psychoanalytic writers such as Ogden (1992) and Sandler (1993) in their descriptions of projective identification. Sandler describes how the client provokes, prods, and manipulates the therapist. He describes how the client can "impose an interaction, an inter-relationship, between themselves and their therapists" (p. 44). Thus, the therapist is unconsciously drawn into an intersubjective engagement. This notion takes us into the heart of the transferential domain, whereby the client's internal object relations come alive in the dyadic relationship.

Secondary Intersubjectivity

Secondary intersubjectivity, which generally develops between 6 and 12 months, requires a greater sophistication in shared affective states and interpersonal understanding. The infant understands (m)other's intention and at the same time (on the basis of shared meaning and understanding) can enhance this to include sharing a sense of a third mediating object or person. The interaction can, from this point, begin to extend its topics to include joint action and joint attention. At this stage, infants begin to understand that events and objects in the world can be shared in the experience of two people; therefore, the infant can turn his or her attention to things other than the immediate interaction itself.

Although the focus of this article is on the immediate nonverbal transactions from mainly primary intersubjective interaction (see vignette to follow), it is useful at this point to consider some differences between primary and secondary intersubjective relating. The emergence of the ability to relate at a secondary intersubjective level can be construed as a developmental achievement in itself. In keeping with the notion of the "dyadic origin of mind" (Trevarthen and Stern), it would seem that both primary and secondary relational experiences are developmental in nature. In everyday interaction, these two types of intersubjective ability are interrelated in terms of processing and will often overlap, with the differences between them sometimes subtle and blurred. For example, this might be the case within secondary intersubjective interactions, with no overt primary intersubjective exchanges in the field, when there is the underlying reality of unconscious-type primary intersubjective processing occurring concurrently in at least a regulatory manner. We are postulating that the qualitative differences between the direct me/thee affective interaction of primary intersubjectivity and secondary-type intersubjective interactions will lead to different levels of self-construction and reconstruction, and that these differences are of value for practitioners to comprehend and utilize.

As mentioned earlier, secondary intersubjective interaction extends to topics that involve a third mediating object or person and includes joint action and joint attention. However, prior to the development of secondary intersubjectivity (and throughout the life span), primary intersubjective abilities are our main route to meeting the mind of the other in a direct sense. This makes sense in terms of the developmental requirement of the infant to become, to acquire a sense of self from which it can then go on to further develop, interpret, and function.

Ultimately, in its different forms, secondary intersubjective relating—by its defining feature of the participants focusing joint attention on a subject outside of the immediate interpersonal exchange—moves us away from a me/thee direct experience and, as such, will not have the same core-self-affecting impact as the more purely self-affecting primary process. To use Stern's (1985, p. 97) concept of Representations of Interactions that have been Generalized (RIGs), we suggest that those constructed from primary and secondary intersubjective experiences will, in essence, differ.

To help illustrate this point, it is useful to think of the particular quality of primary intersubjectivity shaped by the immediacy of interactions (such as attunement or disruptions in attunement) and through which a knowing of the other and self emerges that is particular to this type of meeting of minds. These engagements are geared toward knowing the other and self directly and intimately, and they foster self-constructive events such as identification and mimicry at a level that impacts directly on our core self-experience.

In practice, it can be seen from transactions such as, for example, when a client says, "I was angry with my mother when she" (joint attention on a subject) or "I was angry at you last week" (joint attention at a more subtle level) that while both of these interactions lead us into an understanding of the other's experience and can, indeed, enhance our understanding of each other, they are different in quality from, say, the experience of being in a space with a client in which the person is being loving or furious in the here and now with you. The latter interpersonal events resonate quite differently within us, and hence our knowing of and response to the other at this level is quite different in quality. The knowing of self and other that emerges from these differing intersubjective relational experiences will thus differ. We postulate that this difference will be at the core of the emerging methodology and practice that attempts to facilitate transformation of the core sense of self.

The intensity as to which primary or secondary intersubjective encounters are being enacted between any two subjectivities also needs to be taken into account when considering these matters. It can take passion to heat up a relationship, and as selves take shape within relationship, these passionate exchanges are more likely to provide the heat required to foster fluidity of self. Using this analogy, it is useful to view feelings between therapist and client—such as love, sadness, or fury—as passionate exchanges, and if shied away from, potential self-constructive opportunities may be missed.

Bateson (1972), Brazelton (Brazelton & Cramer, 1991; Brazelton et al., 1975), Fivas-Depeursinge (1991), Sylvester-Bradley (as cited in Miell & Dallos, 1996), and Watzlawick (1963) all come to varying conclusions that testify to the significance of intersubjective relatedness in the realms of preverbal communication, with a focus on breathing and facial and body gestures between infant and caretaker and the evidence of unconscious projection of feelings of anxiety and frustration onto the child.

Thus, infant research shows the complexity of the dialogic exchange and suggests a complex, preverbal, and intelligent infant. It shows that learning, intellectual and emotional development, and a sense of self evolve out of complex interrelational patterns that are coconstructed between infant and caretaker and can be understood as intersubjective relatedness. This domain continues throughout life.

To summarize, the crucial components of intersubjectivity that have emerged from this discussion so far include the following:

It is an existential given.

It is a process of mutuality that is sometimes asymmetrical; in other words, mutuality does not imply equality.

It is the overlap of two minds, in a shared state of being, as in a meeting of minds in the in-between space that is sometimes described as a type of third subjectivity.

It involves both primary and secondary intersubjective relating, which are potentially self-constructive in nature, although they have qualities that impact on different parts of the domains of self.

It is a developmental achievement that involves the ability to recognize the existence of another subjectivity as described earlier in the shared focus idea of secondary intersubjectivity.

Most importantly, and continuing in the relational tradition within transactional analysis, it immediately becomes clear that the notion of pathology residing in the client alone is a reductionistic and clinically unhelpful notion. Instead, the theory of intersubjectivity emphasizes the emotional environment—the intersubjective conditions—and requires us to analyze why and how experience is organized within the client, between client and therapist, and within the therapist.

While none of our clients are infants (although some of us do work with children, of course), what is the implication of infant research for psychotherapy with both adults and children? The research simply shows that the optimal development of human beings involves nonverbal intersubjective transactions and that this process is central to how a sense of self develops, is sustained, and evolves toward its intellectual and emotional potential. These interactional patterns continue developing into adulthood as described by Stern's (1985) domains of the self. Thus, the nonverbal aspect of communication influences an ongoing development of self. It follows that an analysis of the emergent nonverbal transactional patterns between therapist and client will reveal a picture of the client's sense of self and the extent to which this sense is ruptured or distorted.

Implications for Transactional Analysis

So what does this mean in relation to current transactional analysis theory and practice? We think it important that we as transactional analysts take into consideration these developmentally crucial nonverbal and unconscious interactions, interactions in which a different type of knowing develops. For instance, the aforementioned developmental research alters our understanding of the Adult ego state. While it is true that we all have the capacity to think, it is now clear that thinking is more than cognitive symbolic thought. The development of the ability to think is contingent, at least in part, on complex relational experiences, which implicates the notion of a shared mind. The "reflexive functions" described by Diamond and Marrone (2003, pp. 129–130), which are coconstructed within the primary intersubjective relational experience, are nonsymbolic in nature and are essential to and underlie development of what we would describe as Adult abilities (e.g., symbolic thinking, here-and-now reasoning, and understanding of self and other as having separate subjectivities). We postulate that what we would term "Adult capacities" emerge in part from affective interaction and as such are relationally constructed. Since we are continually forming and reforming, we wonder if Adult processing may be more helpfully constituted as an integration of conscious, unconscious, verbal, and nonverbal experience and relating in the here and now. In our view, this offers a fuller psychological and emotional sense of the Adult ego state.

Clearly, this has implications for transactional analysis theory and practice. To highlight this, we use the example of a traditional transactional analysis intervention with clients who have a disorder of the self. It is typical to describe such therapy in terms of first working with the client to help him or her to develop a strong Adult before going on to deconfusion work. We are not disagreeing with the essence of this intervention, but we do disagree with the theory and methodology currently employed by transactional analysts to inform the "how to" develop Adult abilities. We postulate that by setting up conditions conducive to the emergence of underlying reflexive capacities (e.g., holding, containment, empathic experiences, and relational experiences, all "scaffolded" within the primary intersubjective exchange), clients defined as self-disordered will be served most effectively. In a sense, the Adult is created from a combination of both bottom-up and top-down processing. This way of thinking about the development of the Adult is highlighted by the use of the introjective and transformational transferences (Hargaden & Sills, 2002), which lead to two types of transferential relationships based on the qualitites just described.

Following from this, we can begin to question the notion of symbiosis within an intersubjective frame that includes the notion of a shared mind. From there, we ask ourselves the question, "Is normal here-and-now appropriate behavior more a complex mix of interconnectedness within conscious and unconscious processing?" We think so and thus suggest that concepts such as dependency and pathology require more careful definition.

For instance, there are two common meanings given to games. One is that we play games to acquire strokes and reinforce script beliefs or life position; the other is that at a level of unconscious processing, games are an attempt, through projection, to recreate a scene with the hope of a more satisfactory outcome (as in transference). Games and transference, viewed from an intersubjective perspective, however, offer another viewpoint, one that involves a wider, more complex system of intersubjective relating. In short, the meanings given to games, symbiosis, and transference were set within a context in which research tended to view the self as separate. If transactional analysis is to utilize current research into the human condition, it will have to address the issue of giving new meanings to these concepts, ones that are in relation to a self that is interconnected throughout the life span. By responding differently to these phenomena, we can enter the space our clients direct us to and be more fully with them in order to help elaborate and process their development within a "scaffolded" encounter.

A simple example of a current transactional analysis intervention causing relational disruption can be seen in the practice of discount assessment and the subsequent crossing of game transactions. If a client, for instance, is developmentally bereft of relational experiences in which his or her reflexive potentials (nonsymbolic and symbolic) would have otherwise emerged in the context of attachment to an other, therapists can, by crossing the transactions, both close down avenues for transformation and also inadvertently make inaccurate assumptions based on their client's behavior. Assumptions made about clients' motivation—for instance, that they are discounting reality so as to remain in the game to collect a payoff and further their script—whether accurate or not, can lead to a further "missing" of those clients and harmful disruption of the intersubjective process (harmful in the sense of foreclosing meaning). We may then be unwittingly persecuting "stuck" clients when they have not yet developed the underlying reflexive abilities required to be able to respond in what we term "Adult."

By utilizing the intersubjective position, we can both understand more completely just what is happening relationally between client and therapist and come to recognize the subjectivity of the therapist as central to the therapeutic encounter. We do this by:

Noticing our direct experience of being with the client, for instance, engaging internally with our own disruptions and distortions that become particularly prevalent with a particular client

Being conscious of our own sense of self so that we do not enact our hurts and injuries but are conscious that we are perhaps being pulled into doing so

Being conscious of how we are impacting the intersubjective experience so that we recognize how our tiny movements (e.g., flickering eyes and tone of voice) may well betray our better intentions

Being available to coconstruct new relational experience, to make sense of emerging data so that even if the client is not quite ready, we are at least available to cothink or to suggest a way of cothinking our way through the emergent intersubjective processes

By engaging with the client in these ways, we can more competently and effectively work with the unconscious processes existing between us.

Clinical Practice: A Therapist's Subjective

Experience

The following piece is a fictionalized example based on clinical experience (Hargaden, 2004); we present it here to describe the intersubjective transferential interaction in minute detail, as though under a "feelings" microscope.

I hear the client's words and observe that she is talking about herself in harsh tones. I think about the internalized persecutory Parent, and I also think about the controlled and unhappy Child-like feelings. Then I think: impasse. Initially, I feel harangued by her and shift about uncomfortably in my chair. Part of me wishes she would go away. I feel quite pressured to sort something out, or is it that I feel pressure to shut her up and that sorting something out might make this noise go away?

As I notice these feelings and thoughts within me, I want to say, "Stop, let's look at these problems. I'm sure they can be worked out. I'm sure you don't have to go to such lengths to try and get everything done." But I decide to hold my feelings for the moment. I am not sure what is going on and I feel the need to wait for a while. I feel as though I am being induced into a mood but I don't know what it is, so I stay with the silent holding, thinking that I may foreclose on something if I step in too soon. I notice her face, drawn and anxious, eyes darting rapidly around the room. I feel anxious and want to solve the problem. Maybe I could suggest that she talk to her internal objects through two-chair work and shift some of the energy away from me!

Meanwhile, I have not said a word to interrupt her, and her tone becomes more agitated as she speaks even more rapidly. I am reminded of gunfire. I feel the presence of someone in the room shooting words at me, and I feel attacked and want to cry. I feel as though I am a little girl and someone is shouting at me to do something and I don't know what it is. I feel a vague sense of this having happened to me, and then I begin to feel sad and that I want to weep, although the client does not seem sad at all.

Intuitively now, I know she must be feeling absolutely dreadful, and so I eventually manage to "get hold of her eyes" with my eyes, and I say, "You seem sad today." I feel tender, so my voice is soft and concerned in tone, which contrasts with the harshness of her tone and words. There is a stunned silence, and I feel some relief. Then she weeps and weeps and weeps, and eventually together she and I make sense of it all—mostly her—with me nodding and adding some thoughts along the way based on script and structural analytic interpretations.

In this brief vignette, the emphasis is on nonverbal communication. The two people in the room are in an implicit intersubjective relationship. Although the client is talking at the therapist, there is also another level of relatedness that comes into the therapist's consciousness as she recognizes that she feels attacked by the words, which sound like "gunfire." She wonders if this is what the client feels toward herself.

Many therapists will recognize how much patience and self-discipline it takes to work in this intersubjective frame. The therapist's subjectivity and the subsequent focus of the therapist's and client's attention within the therapeutic encounter become the key to effective therapy. The extent to which therapists allow themselves to be penetrated by clients' affective states and meanings, involving them in an active emotional dynamic, will be a more accurate marker of the progress of therapy than theoretical explanations.

In the case example, the therapist initially tried to resist the penetration of the client's feelings of desperation and sadness. The therapist wanted to eagerly point out the "way" to her client, which could be understood as empathizing with the "defensive self." However, the relational process is the opposite of an intentional one; it is, in essence, a journey involving an uncertainty of destination but a certainty of emotional upheaval and disturbance in both client and therapist. This process leads to an elaboration on, or transformation of, experience of self, other, and the world, as in the transformational transference described by Hargaden and Sills (2002). Only when the therapist was willing for her own ego needs to become subservient to the therapeutic task of listening with heightened attunement to the feelings of isolation, desperation, and sadness gradually emerging within herself could she be of any use to her client. This leads to a more self-constructive, empathic experience, one that is aligned to a more "real self" position, which we postulate is the crucible for core self-transformation.

It has been commonly observed that no psychic change will occur in the client unless the therapist, too, is changed emotionally in some way. In the example, the therapist had to let go of her enthusiasm for changing her client and instead make herself engage with her client differently. In those moments she knew herself and her client in a different way, and in the process the client came to know herself through the eyes and feelings of the therapist.

The use of the therapist's face is central to nonverbal communication. Eigen (1993) observed that "the centrality of the human face as symbolic of personality permeates the fabric of human experience" (p. 49). He suggested that the human face is the most important "organizing principle in the field of meaning" (p. 56). By seeking to find the client's eyes, the therapist in the vignette is providing a type of emotional scaffolding within which the client can feel held and, to a certain extent, be led into a connection with her self. The therapist leads the way with her nonverbal gestures before naming the feeling. The client's feelings change from anger, irritation, and frustration into sadness when she sees acceptance of her vulnerable sense of self in the therapist's eyes and hears it in the therapist's tone of voice in ways she has longed for but feels simultaneously ashamed of. As she starts to change, the client is more able to think as the word "sad" reaches her, and in a moment of recognition, she begins to weep.

We get a sense here of how the client is using the therapist as a transforming object through being offered the experience of staying within the immediate to and fro of the relationship, the realm of primary intersubjectivity and core self-experience. Initially, in a nonverbal, presymbolic state in which the psychological exchange occurs at a feeling level, therapist and client are involved in negotiating shared meaning through the unconscious transferring of emotional states, that is, through the shared third subjective space as postulated by Trevarthen. This process segues into a secondary intersubjective phase in the sense that they both have their joint attention on the subject of the client's distress. The client's thinking emerges in the interactional context as in cothinking referred to earlier. By changing the environment for the client through tone, gesture, and facial expression, the therapist enables the client to change and eventually use language to make further changes in her thinking, reflecting as she did on her earlier state of distress. Furthermore, her narrative in terms of how she understood herself changed from thinking about herself harshly and critically to a more thoughtful account of the origins of her distress. Thus, thinking, making sense, and bringing about script changes can be seen to be directly linked to the prior process of nonverbal engagement and the experience of shared minds.

We can see from infant research that parts of the self become buried early on, and some parts may never develop at all when there have been significant failures in parenting. The counterscripted self, as depicted by Hargaden and Sills (2002) in the development of a defensive sense of A_1, can be identified by the client's unconscious attempts to find influence within the therapeutic relationship. Clients will do so in a manner reflecting the early coconstructed relational patterns that emerged within their original relational matrix. These patterns will have originally allowed them to feel a sense of mutuality or control within their early relational context. These patterns are generally a rich source of data for the therapist and can often be identified through analysis of unconscious processes, such as countertransference. Methods such as questioning ourselves in an ongoing way—for example, "What is the client trying to get me to do?"—can often help bring into awareness these unconscious attempts at controlling the relational experience. However, if these processes go unnoticed, they can, over time, have a negative effect on the therapy and maybe even on the therapist's psyche in terms of our unconsciously making adjustments toward manipulative relational patterns.

In the vignette, the therapist originally felt great pressure to respond practically, which she resisted with difficulty in a fashion similar to the client's original relational experience with her mother. The therapist recognized how she had been pulled to repeat the pattern and that part of her had wanted to avoid the psychic isolation and pain that her client was wanting her to understand through unconscious processing. The pressure to repeat the pattern can be very strongly felt, as it was in this case, where the client's needs to be seen, heard, and even found emotionally were distorted and expressed through the defenses of script and game enactments (e.g., in presenting the problem as a practical one for which she did not have a solution). Instead, the therapist had to forego her own defense against feeling. Not only was she impacted by her client, but in the process she felt emotionally changed when a distant sense emerged within her of having felt persecuted, along with a critical dismissing of herself in a persecutory fashion, as just a victim in her own relational past/history. In feeling empathy for her client, the therapist felt empathy for that isolated self state that had emerged into consciousness in the work, and in those moments she too was changed.

In a sense, at the end of the therapeutic encounter, the outcome for therapist and client in terms of self was that they both ended up "part me part you." The client found herself through the therapist, as in projective transference, and then through the therapist in a different way, as in introjective transference. She constructed a new part of herself in response to her newly recovered parts. In short, this case example shows how we are constantly finding old and recreating new selves within here-and-now relational experiences.

The intersubjective process, of course, carries with it the potential for all types of engagement that are not so identifiably empathic, such as disruptive or adversarial connections. For example, a client who felt she had to be seen as a highly fragile, sensitive person was shocked when the therapist engaged with her in a robust and potentially discordant manner. The therapist's use of her subjectivity as a type of divining rod led her toward a truer self, hidden under the client's compensatory A_1 presentation, in which she was highly anxious to be seen in a stereotypically feminine way.

The therapist may feel obliged or pressured to engage with the client's scripted self and bypass, yet again, the underlying, unseen, unrecognized, and as yet undeveloped self. The extent to which we do this and at the same allow for the recovery of an emergent sense of true self (referred to by Stern [1985] as the seat of all our creativity) is linked to the skills and consciousness of the therapist. Maybe therapy at its best and most satisfying is about the uncovering of this domain, in which lies our core sense of creativity. The use of poetry, story, and choice of words are often clues to the subjective nonverbal experience. For example, if a therapist refers to her "tender" feelings toward a client, she immediately creates a different type of environment than if she uses the word "fondness." But perhaps the most important aspect of the verbal domain lies in how the client finds the words to tell her own story.

Therapists are not mothers, but we are inevitably endowed with the possibilities and potential symbolized in the great mother archetype: the giver of life, the capacity for genuine love, and the container of hope. These qualities are not gender specific, but they can be generated within the therapeutic atmosphere and can be understood as metaphors for psychic rebirth. Thus, the here-and-now relationship between therapist and client becomes a highly charged unity of potential and possibility for psychological transformation of both client and therapist.

Conclusion

Infant research offers compelling evidence for the significance of intersubjectivity in human connectedness. Stern (1985) has shown how the nonverbal domains of self continue throughout our lives. There is, therefore, a clinical imperative to engage with the nonverbal interactive field of transactions. The nonverbal is a way we both consciously and unconsciously convey our sense of self, regulate our sense of self through interaction with another, and reconstruct our sense of self in a conscious and unconscious way within relational experiences. As therapists, our job is to focus on, understand, and utilize these processes in an effort to understand more fully our transformational role within the client's psyche, thus leaving less to chance. Our job is paradoxically to let go of theory and become our "self," to develop a sensibility that seeks to engage with clients as though on a journey of discovery for ourselves as well as for them. From the intersubjective perspective, we expect our emotional history to become implicated in the client's journey with a view to furthering the client's psychological health and, in the process, find that once again, we are also changed.

Furthermore, a theory of intersubjectivity provides the conceptual building blocks by which we can understand the unconscious process. As Aron (2001) writes,

> Today, in the sciences and across all disciplinary pursuits, the polarization of subjectivity and objectivity has been questioned, the subjectivity of the investigator has been incorporated into disciplinary methodologies, and we have begun to investigate the nature and development of intersubjectivity. (p. 64)

Theories of intersubjectivity provide transactional analysts with new and interesting ways of conceptualizing the analysis of transactions and deepen further the transferential matrix and development of self suggested in the relational work of Hargaden and Sills (2002).

Finally, by concentrating on the nonverbal domain of relatedness, we are by no means excluding the significance of the verbal domain. It is, however, clinically important to recognize that because language can so easily become the dominant discourse of meaning, much will be lost if we fail to give careful attention to the nonverbal interactions that take us into the heart of the person's experience of self.

REFLECTIONS

This chapter focuses on one moment in time in a therapy, which the authors use to analyse developmental perspectives in theoretical depth. The inspiration for the article began with a session I had with a client, recounted in the article, which coincided with a supervision group I was leading which consisted of eight senior practitioners. I presented my case study as a prompt for a group discussion about non-verbal intersubjectivity. This began a series of discussions between Brian Fenton, a group member, and myself. It was time for us to take a deeper dive into the theory of intersubjectivity of the non-verbal domain.

Brian had a wealth of knowledge from his open university course completed some years previously, and introduced me to the ideas of Trevarthen and Vysogotsky. We are careful in the chapter to make links with Berne's theories but, clearly, as with the relational turn, we are moving in a direction far away from behavioural and cognitive theory beloved by the classical school of TA with its emphasis upon individuality and separate minds. It is now possible to match the findings of these developmental psychiatrists, Trevarthen and Vysogotsky, with our understanding of the right hemisphere of the mind, Damasio, McGilchrist, and Schore. Vysgotsky (1896–1934), a soviet psychiatrist, emphasised the shared nature of our seemingly individual minds and selves. He proposed that emotional affective states are shared before mental states that refer to objects outside of the dyad. Trevarthan, a developmental psychologist, argued that intersubjectivity exists as a human capacity. Their work, alongside others such as Diamond and Marrone, foreshadowed the neuroscientific evidentce that the mother's mind is linked to the baby's mind by the placenta; that the first two years of life of the baby are formed through nonverbal, proto conversations that are emotional in tone; that the source of our subjectivity is nonverbal and resplendent in emotional, intuitive experiences that are full of imagery and may never be made fully conscious. In the same way what is in the mind of the therapist, known and unknown will impact the client and vice versa. Out of this complex mix, we will find the ingredients of the unconscious.

Chapter 2

The Role of the Imagination in an Analysis of Unconscious Relatedness

Helena Hargaden

The impetus for writing this chapter was my passion for discovering the multilayered meanings inherent in the clinical encounter. In the following case study, divided into two parts, I explore how the use of the imagination, reflection, and therapeutic congruence offer serious methods of analysis enabling us to understand our work more creatively. The following theoretical perspectives are discussed as a way of illuminating these processes: the theory of enactments (Bromberg, 2006; Stuthridge, 2012), Bion's (1959) theory of reverie, the theory of the third (Benjamin, 2004; Gerson, 2004), Jung's (1991) theory of archetypes, and scientific paradigms of the mind (Damasio, 1999; Schore, 2003/2012). This chapter expands on the relational understanding of projective identification described in the domains of transference, with particular focus on the transformational transference (Hargaden & Sills, 2002).

Part One: Marianne—In the Beginning

When Marianne came into therapy, she was 34. She was a tall, slender woman, stylishly dressed, and a highly achieving professional in the field of science. Initially, we talked about her current situation as a single parent with an unsupportive male ex-partner whom she experienced as vindictive and unable to parent their young daughter with any consistency. Early in the therapy, Marianne made some decisions to help her disentangle herself from him and secure economic security for herself and her daughter. Feeling safer and more assured, she began to talk about her childhood. Her background is complex, and her relationship with her mother and siblings would make an interesting study. However, here I will concentrate on Marianne's experience with her father as this is related to the two parts of this chapter.

When Marianne first described her father's brutal treatment of her (which was both physical and mental), I would become indignant, expressing a type of furious empathy with her childhood experience. Instead of feeling understood, Marianne had felt under threat, which initially puzzled me.

DOI: 10.4324/9781032266237-3

At such times, I felt as if I were mentally wrestling with her internalized subjugating father, trying to free the Child from his malevolent influence on her. The most striking consequence of his hold on her manifest itself in excoriating self-criticism. "Sorry" was a frequently used word that was most confusing because it was unclear what Marianne was apologizing for. I learned that the word "sorry" seemed to mean: "Sorry I exist. Sorry that I have an opinion. Sorry that I might be hurting someone with my very presence. Sorry that you might find me difficult."

However, there was also a defiant quality to the way Marianne said "sorry," as though she was angry that she had to apologize. I found myself being very direct and blunt, matching her negative view of herself with a type of maternal ferocity. I tried to show empathy with the vulnerable child who had been under continuous malicious threats from her father. But Marianne could not tolerate thinking about her vulnerability, and so our interactions tumbled over each other, as though competing for space. Both of us lacked genuine confidence in ourselves and each other. It was as if we needed to make our points, make ourselves heard, while both failing to hear the other. We were embroiled in an enactment.

There is clearly a link with games theory to be made here, and for those wishing for a more definitive discussion of the similarities and differences between games and enactments, I recommend Novak's (2015) excellent article on the subject. Here I will concentrate only on the theory of enactments.

An Enactment

An enactment is the acting out, in the interpersonal field between therapist and client, of dissociated aspects of their psyches. Bromberg (2006) described an enactment as a rupture in the therapeutic relationship that allows dissociated material to emerge between therapist and client. Stuthridge (2012) viewed enactments in therapy as an opportunity "to discover the lost parts of oneself for both client and therapist" (p. 12). Enactments are, therefore, a means by which unconscious material can emerge in the therapy.

In the enactment with Marianne, I felt that I was up against an implacable force that had entered the space between us, one that left no room for reflection, feeling, or empathy. After such sessions, I felt winded. What had happened? I struggled to find my mind. Although I was able to think theoretically about Marianne's need for defense systems, I was emotionally blank and disconnected from any more meaningful reflections. My phenomenological experience during these sessions manifested itself in an odd bodily reaction in which I felt as though air was being pumped into me followed by a sensation of bursting open. I was unable to hold the process. There was no container, nothing but a sense of flying rubbish in which thoughts, feelings, and ideas were detonated and destroyed. I criticized myself for arguing with her, for not finding more nuanced ways to get at the points I thought should be made, the interpretations I knew had to be offered, the explanations I insisted on.

When I began to recognize that we were in an enactment, I was able to ask myself some questions: Why were my interventions so insistent and forceful? Why did I persist? Insist? Try harder? Viewing my countertransference through a personal lens, I could see I might still be trying to heal my mother. There seemed to be something seductive about Marianne's suffering that resonated with a desperate Child state in me from the past, who, if she had had the words, would have screamed, "No need to carry on being a Victim."

As Stuthridge (2012) pointed out, the dissociation occurs in both therapist and client; it is a form of unconscious relatedness. The dissociated part of me was linked to the unconscious projection of my mother onto Marianne. My mother had had a brutal father. Although I had not consciously understood that as a child, I had tried to compensate for her suffering at the same time that I felt frustrated that all my efforts were wasted because she always sank back into her Victimhood. This was also an example of how transgenerational trauma (Hargaden, 2013b; Wallfisch, 2013) moves unconsciously from one generation to another. My grandfather's war traumas had transmitted themselves through a violent brutality he showed toward my mother, whom I have come to believe he also envied because of her love of books and introverted temperament. In the following discussion, it will become clear how her dissociated transgenerational trauma affected Marianne and also shaped our enacted dialogue. In part two, the dissociated trauma emerges as a viseral experience in the room between us.

When I eventually moved out of the enactment by developing a cognitive understanding of the process I was in with Marianne, I was able to contain my reactions more carefully. However, it was only when I fell into a reverie that the emotional way out of our impasse and the meaning of the enactment became clearer.

Using the Third as a Way Out of the Impasse

For those not familiar with the theory of *the third,* it has its roots in Freud's (1899/1953) theory of the Oedipus complex. The theory of the third is a modern and more expanded way of thinking about the function of the father, which is to interrupt the symbiosis between mother and child as part of the healthy development of the self. The third refers to this symbolic father, now translated into a theory of thirds that describes a process by which the therapeutic dyad is interrupted and altered by a third force. Gerson (2004) referred to the creation of a triangular symbolic space that can emerge from a collision of polarities in which a third way is formed. What he meant is that the therapist needs to find a part of her that both participates in the polarity but at the same time is able to find a corner of her mind to reflect on what is going on. It is this corner of the therapist's mind that is called the third. It is as if a third person is introduced into the therapeutic dyad. In this way, the third functions as a symbol for finding a way out of the binary of the therapeutic relationship.

Once you begin considering thirds in this way, you can have as many thirds as you can think of. For instance, Gerson (2004) suggested three categories of potential thirds: developmental, cultural, and relational. The clinical benefits of thinking about thirds are many, one of which is to enable the members of a therapeutic couple to find their way out of binary processes using the third as a symbol (in whatever category).

The Emergence of the Third in the Therapy With Marianne

The third emerged with Marianne in the middle of yet another heated interpersonal dynamic one day. I became aware of a light bouncing off the white shutters in front of the window. It felt almost sunny, although the day was grey. With the light, a feeling of softness came into the room. I rubbed my hands over the wool of my jumper, an action that I found soothing and that helped me to fall quiet. It became possible to feel some emotional warmth and to take time to reflect.

My Reflections on the Making of a Subjugating Father

In that session with Marianne, I found myself musing on my work with two male clients with whom I have been working, both over a period of 18 years. These men had been to high-ranking boarding schools. I had learned not only concrete knowledge of how these institutions worked but had witnessed, and at times absorbed, the traumatic experience each had suffered in the British boarding school system (both came to me three times a week for many years). The material conditions were akin to a type of penal servitude. Heating, food, and beds were normally kept to minimal standards. Any expression of vulnerability occasioned severe humiliation, disgust, and punishment (Schaverin, 2015). The reasoning behind such institutionalized torture was apparently to make men who would fight for, and defend, the British Empire. This was how the British stiff upper lip was created. In thinking about my male clients, and the depth of suffering they had endured (one had been sent to school at the age of four), I began to reflect on Marianne's father, who had also gone to boarding school. I used my reflections to open up a conversation with Marianne about what she knew of her father's background.

The Destruction of the Maternal

Listening to Marianne, it became clear that her father had been raised in conditions of severe maternal deprivation. He had been separated from his mother at an early age and thrown into the boarding school environment where empathy and maternal warmth were denigrated, derided, and destroyed. I began to understand why my every effort to develop a maternal containing presence had been attacked. My phenomenological experience of mindlessness, of bursting open, of feeling unable to contain, had mirrored how the maternal container had cracked in her father's original experience, separated from his mother at an early age. As I shared my reflections about the nature of boarding schools and their effects on young boys, both Marianne and I began to see her father differently. She had internalized an experience of her father as a demonic monster who ruled his family with brutal authoritarianism, but as we reflected on the meanings inherent in her father's experience, her view of him began to change. Her father emerged in our conversation as a rather tragic figure, a sad person who had been weakened rather than strengthened by his experiences of maternal deprivation. In viewing her father this way, we began to reflect together that his abuse of Marianne was more mindless than personal, that it revealed much more about him than her.

However, there is a tipping point over which you do not go as a therapist, where sympathy for the parent starts to outweigh the damage they have inflicted. Together Marianne and I began to understand the extent of her father's traumatic legacy and how it had shaped her internal world and, indeed, our dialogue and therapeutic interactions. Despite his mindless brutality, she had stood up to her father, and, although terrified, she had fought him on the battlefront of ideas. Paradoxically, she also sought to protect him, intuitively sensing his vulnerability. Thinking together about these dynamics, we began to recognize that his expressed hatred of her was, at times, probably an expression of envy for her spirit of defiance against subjugation, for showing a type of courage and strength that had long since been knocked out of him. Also, we thought, he had envied her natural inclination to try to nurture him, something he both wanted but despised. It was through these conversations that Marianne began to take back the power she had invested in him, to see him for what he was, and to begin a journey toward owning her own agency.

From this perspective, we both began to understand why the emergence of trust and love in the therapy, signified by my ferocious empathy, was so threatening. She was enabled to feel the extent of her desolation and despair and to be more open to the vulnerable self that emerged between the two of us. She moved out of the Victim position (Karpman, 1968) and began to see cause for a legitimate sorrow for the child who had been wounded by a traumatizing narcissistic father (Shaw, 2014).

The cumulative effect of these sessions paved the way for a nonlinear therapeutic process that I will describe in part two of this chapter. As Marianne became more trusting of me and more open to her feeling world, I was able to feel the strength of being secure in not knowing (Bachelard, 1958/1994) and more able to listen to the unconscious.

To get to this point in the therapy, it was crucial to recognize the enactment, to take time to reflect on my feelings and be open to my introspection. This was the method by which a third way emerged that deepened the therapeutic conversation in the ways I will now describe.

Part Two: Marianne on the Couch

Capturing the nuances and many metaphorical meanings of a clinical encounter is quite a challenge. According to Naiburg (2015), "One of your challenges as a clinical writer is to translate analytic and qualitative experience and the poetry of what we do (and feel and intuit …) with our patients into prose, knowing how inadequate any translation might be" (p. 10). Naiburg's notion chimes with Ogden (2004), who wrote, "An analytic experience—like all other experiences, does not come to us in words. An analytic experience cannot be told or written; an experience is what it is" (p. 16).

Naiburg's and Ogden's ideas are also reflected in the work of Daniel Stern (1985) when he described our first sense of self as the emergent sense of self, the seat of our creativity, which is nonverbal. In Stern's domains of the self, he suggested that the verbal self often alienates us from the emergent self. The philosopher and psychoanalyst Julia Kristever (1969/1980) described this earliest sense of self as the *semiotic*. She referred to Lacan's theory that the use of language signifies "the father," who interrupts the symbiosis between mother and child. Kristever argued that it is through the language of the father that we learn to be ashamed, not only of our bodies (associated as they are with the maternal function) but of our fundamental core relational experience, needs, and sense of this semiotic self.

How then to think about, understand, and write about clinical experiences that involve the semiotic, the nonverbal? We need to find a different language because the language of logic, the language of the father, cannot adequately describe the language of the unconscious mind and the multifaceted experience of psychotherapy.

Naiburg and Ogden spoke to the essence of the challenge to put the intensity of multifaceted experience into language. This is of central importance for psychotherapy because the nature of trauma means it has not been metabolized or mentalized (Fonagy & Target, 1998) but is often somatized. The scientific basis for thinking about different types of thinking and language is supported by neuroscience (Damasio, 1999; Schore, 2003/ 2012). Thus, trauma cannot be dealt with through cognitive means.

In the case study described here, reverie was used as a channel through which to retrieve traumatic experience. Bion (1959) thought that reverie was a crucial variable in the creation of an analytic process that promotes therapeutic action through learning from experience. "An understanding mother is able to experience the feeling of dread, that this baby was striving to deal with by projective identification, and yet retain a balanced outlook" (p. 313). Bion called this ability the *alpha function* in the mother, that is, she is someone who can pick up the projective identification and make emotional meaning out of it. He thought that the therapist's alpha function capacity provided a necessary stimulus for the patient, encouraging a process of transformation that makes it possible to experience that which could not be tolerated or approached before. In other words, therapists must allow themselves to delve into the area of the unknown, to go with the flow of the unconscious, to use their imaginations and listen to themselves. These self-states are necessary to allow for the unspeakable to emerge and then to find different words in which to speak about it. In the following account, reverie becomes a significant method by which that is achieved.

A Paradigm of the Mind

Neurological research (Damasio, 1999; Schore, 2003/2012) has shown that the brain is capable of two kinds of thinking: One is linear and logical, the other is nonlinear. The left hemisphere of the brain is associated with syntactical speech, and the right hemisphere is associated with emotional and musical expression. Trauma, which exists in the unconscious or is usually experienced primarily nonverbally, cannot be dealt with through cognitive means. The language of logic cannot describe the language of the nonlinear unconscious mind.

From a metaphorical perspective, Jung (1991) referred to the linear and logical part of the psyche as the *masculine archetype*. He described the poetic, nonlinear part of the psyche as the *feminine archetype*. Jung's terms have proved controversial over the years because they have sometimes been thought to be stereotyping of gender.

However, I think such criticism misinterprets what Jung meant. I use the terms "feminine" and "masculine" for two reasons. One is that Jung (1991) greatly valued the feminine, by which he did not mean gender but an archetypal, primitive mental image inherent in the collective unconscious. The feminine archetype refers to a quality of receptivity, of spirit, of an energy that he thought formed the core of the unconscious process. The second reason I find Jung's paradigm helpful is because, in his view, the goal of psychotherapy is consciousness, which involves the bringing together of the opposites of masculine and feminine within us. In my view, it enhances our work to be informed by both a scientific and a metaphorical perspective. Logical theoretical clarity gives confidence to the therapist as she or he delves into the mystery and paradox created by metaphor, thus allowing for play, symbol, the tangential, and the unknown: for the discovery of nonlinear unconscious material.

Based on these paradigms of the mind, the challenge for the therapist is to recognize the emergence of nonlinear dynamics or the feminine archetype and to use it as a gateway to finding the elusive language of the unconscious. The difficulty for poets in translating their poetry into prose becomes the same problem for psychotherapists when describing their clinical encounters: how to describe and to find language that does not destroy, spoil, or reduce the layers of metaphorical meaning entwined in experience.

Numinous Moments

The morning light filters through the shutters as, taking off her stylish suede boots and putting her bag neatly next to them, Marianne segues onto the couch where she lies down. The couch is next to a large window that looks out onto the sea at the end of the road. It is windy today. We fall into a silent immersion. I wait. I feel her quietness. It seems to allow for a quietness in me. This way of being together works well for Marianne. When lying on the couch, she is released from feeling scrutinized and judged. This allows her to enter a different psychological space, a place that allows for the discovery of other selves. I too feel released from an experience often evoked by her of having to make sense of things. Instead, I have a feeling best described as a release from causality. It is as if I move from watching a river to being in the flow of the river.

In this atmosphere, nonlinear dynamics can emerge and do so in the following way. I fall into a reverie. The description of the following reverie seems quite long, but in real time it was very brief.

On the wall in front of me is a picture of Lough Allen in Sligo, the Republic of Ireland, home of my ancestors. Today I am drawn to meditating on it for some reason. The lough suggests depth. I imagine a slight wind ruffling the surface of the lough and find myself musing about how my ancestors taught in the Hedge Schools. This was the name used by small bands of teachers who taught the Irish language illegally because it had been banned by the British. For no conscious reason, I begin to imagine hiding in the reeds around the lake, feeling the wind blowing through the grass. I feel some anxiety: Will we be safe from the marauding force of the colonizing army? I am steeped in this imaginative space, although, as I say, only for a few seconds in real time, when I hear Marianne speaking, as though she is in my mind, as if she is part of my reverie. "It is windy today." It is as if we are both in the picture, but her low murmur also draws my attention to some inner feeling state she does not often have time to inhabit in her busy life. Marianne continues speaking from this inner state: "I remember my grandmother's house, it was warm and safe. She lived in the country, in the winter it was cold, windy outside." She trails off. This was where she used to hide from her father. We are in a conversation that is emerging from unconscious self-states—something is opening up and revealing itself to her, to me, to us. I see an image of a hearth and am reminded of Hestia, goddess of the fireside, the "introverted, inwardly focused archetype" (Shinoda-Bolen, 1984, p. 117).

Hestia represents the homemaker, someone who ushers in domestic order. There is a feeling of home, of warmth in the room together with Marianne. The reference to her grandmother also constellates the archetype of the wise old woman. I feel the sense in Marianne of that longing, the need to feel safe and protected from malign forces. Our conversation continues: "My father once attacked me, forcing me against a wall, hitting me. He was furious with me because I had answered him back, had disagreed with him. He told me he would cut my tongue out." My ancestors were hiding from colonial forces, she was hiding in her grandmother's house from a brutal father. We are together, in hiding, safe, immersed in the amniotic sac of the womb. I think of Winnicott's (1953) maternal immersion. Marianne murmurs her feelings. There is trust in me, in us, and I feel that trust. It feels important to be in this moment, not to dissect it with explanation, to deconstruct with interpretation, to penetrate with inquiries. I ponder why I feel like this, as we sit, lie, quietly together. Should I say something of my thinking? Or allow the feeling moments to be? A negative timber creeps into my thoughts. What am I doing? Is this therapeutic? Should I be doing something, pointing something out, making an interpretation, introduce some theory? Again, I fall into a reverie that took place over a few seconds, although it sounds much longer.

Feminization

My mind wanders to a conference I had recently attended that involved a gathering of people from differing modalities who were interested in relational ideas. At the end of the day, about 40 of us gathered in a circle. As usual in these situations, the majority of those attending were women. One of my much loved and esteemed colleagues began to talk of his disquiet at "the feminization" of the profession. To feminize means "to make or become feminine; to develop female characteristics" (*Chambers Dictionary,* 2014, p. 566). Because no one had a dictionary at hand, and because language is often as confusing as it is clarifying, his meaning was not entirely clear.

Previously, I had heard him critique the maternal in psychotherapy practice. His view was that psychotherapy seemed dominated by an excessively maternal attitude that manifests itself in controlling behaviors disguised as nurture. He thought this attitude was an obstacle to navigating through what, in reality, are the psychological shark-infested waters of depth psychotherapy. I had some sympathy with this view and think that nurture can be used to sidestep the pain involved in meeting our demons, in becoming conscious and in more truthfully and honestly finding ourselves. I even wrote an article in which I offered a critique of empathy used in this way (Hargaden, 2013a). However, on this day of the conference, for some mysterious reasons, the impact of his thoughts were received rather negatively by his colleagues. His comments were experienced as gender stereotyping, biased, with the inference that women are annoying and stupid.

Judging from the passionate and disapproving response by female colleagues in the room, I reflected that he had unwittingly invoked the inner critic that so many women carry within themselves, one that tells them they are unlovable, worthless, and stupid.

The Internalized Subjugating Father

Why, though, was I thinking of this event and my colleague's attitude as I sat with Marianne? Why did this man emerge in my imagination as an introjected archetypal subjugating father, the judge who lays down the laws, a type of Godlike figure who defines what is acceptable and appropriate—in this case, what is proper psychotherapy? This imaginary critic was someone who had the attitude of a tyrant, someone who demanded certainty. I hasten to add that my colleague is nothing like that and, in fact, would be terribly offended if he thought that this was how he was perceived. Indeed, he has a powerful capacity to immerse himself in nonlinear dynamics. However, it was the archetype that had been constellated at the conference that now formed in my mind. It was not my colleague who was the tyrant: It was a part of me! As my client and I sat/lay there together, immersed in the feeling of things, I reflected that the part of me that was self-critical of my introspective, more feminine side, might also be a projective identification. That was probably how Marianne felt about herself, about her vulnerability and her femininity. There was certainly plenty in her history with her father to support that view.

At this point, I think it will be clear to you, since I was having these reveries, that I was quiet and contemplative. Such reflections happened quickly, and as I pondered, I heard Marianne's voice, as though out of nowhere, as if in conversation with my unspoken reflections, recalling childhood memories of being viciously attacked both physically and mentally. Nothing would appease her father, it seemed, until she was made a prisoner of his beliefs and ideas and was willing to forgo and sacrifice her subjectivity on the altar of his fatherhood and his need to possess and control her. Marianne was a slender person and had a sensitive, almost fragile sensibility, but she was tough. She had fought her father at every turn, never succumbing entirely to his need to completely possess her mind.

Although I had heard these stories many times before, that day there was a different tone to her recollections. She was more in the experience of what it had felt like. The dissociated self-states of the trauma were making themselves known. Previously, when she had recounted catastrophic events, I had felt angry with her father, which had the effect of making Marianne react defensively. Now, as I listened, I was more in a state of shock, experiencing a strong somatic countertransference in which I felt an almost intolerable sense of my own fragility. In such an imaginative state, linking back to my reverie on the picture, I found myself wondering how easily I might be broken by an invading army, told to succumb to the superior doctrine, forced to forgo my language and religion, that is, be occupied. In the case of the Irish, they had not succumbed. They had been deeply wounded, of course, then went underground, had been divided, shamed, made inferior, and pitied, but many had also grown defiant, quarrelsome, and even violent, as we know.

Similarly, Marianne had fought strenuously against her father, defied his rule, but that meant she had grown strong in a way that was lopsided. She had not been broken, but she was deeply wounded. The violence invoked in her, which is often the case with women, was turned inward against herself through excoriating self-criticism. She had a sharp and argumentative mind; she could hold her ground on any subject. Deep within her, however, was the wound of her vulnerability, her femininity. It was in this way that we both shared a traumatized mind, one hidden in my unconscious that came to the surface stimulated by the picture on the wall. It was a state that mirrored Marianne's experience of male brutality against her body and mind.

How to analyze this process? How to write about this without deconstructing the layers of metaphorical meaning and thereby destroy it by stamping all over the Holy Ground with large theoretical boots? One method of analysis that emerged when writing this chapter was the use of metaphor to illuminate the experience we had.

Pneuma

I have since discovered a Greek word: *pneuma*. Its earliest meaning, in ancient Greek, was "air in motion, breath, wind" (Pneuma, 2016, ¶ 2). A quotation from Anaximenes, an ancient Greek philosopher, says that "just as our soul (*psyche*), being air (*aer*), holds us together, so do breath (*pneuma*) and air (*aer*) encompass the whole world" (¶ 2). Viewed in this way, Marianne's reference to the wind was a powerful expression. Her sotto voce murmuring of "It is windy today" was pregnant with meaning. Her voice, like a whisper, seemed to usher in a different type of energy. The reference to the wind, already in my subliminal imaginative experience stimulated by the picture on the wall, suggested a powerful energy, one that was out of my conscious awareness. Maybe it was this energy that caused me to reflect before speaking, an energy that held me back so I did not invade her with interpretations and explanations. By not doing that, I was implicitly challenging that the only power was in the language of certainty. Power was no longer located only in the conscious mind, in logos: Power was now located in the listening for the meanings that were elusive. Power was in allowing for the experience to speak to us. Power was in Bion's alpha function. Power was in the feminine.

I intuitively knew that if I drew Marianne's attention to any dimension of her experiencing she would too quickly and easily move into her head space, trying to sort it out, understand it, reduce it to the language of logos, a language with which she was articulate and that, to a certain extent, she had used to control her life as a way of coping with her cut-off traumatic experiences. I knew, too, that to draw attention to her evolving emotional dependency on me at that moment would make her withdraw. She would feel too conscious of a sense of weakness that would feel overwhelmingly shameful: She would pull up the drawbridge. The maternal container that had been so lacking in the first part of Marianne's therapy was now emerging in me and between us. Catastrophic experience could now be felt; terror and horror could emerge into a container that was strong enough to keep her/us safe.

As this trauma emerged into the room, the story of the trauma made itself felt in her body and mine, in my reflections, and in the search for language and meaning. In part, perhaps the trauma we experienced was a shared collective trauma related to the denigration of the feminine, the trauma of powerlessness and social repression, and a contempt for the vulnerable, the poetic, the uncertainty of things. I believe that I was both a participant as well as a witness to Marianne's trauma and the denigration of her as a person and maybe as a woman.

The Thirds

To illuminate these numinous moments, it is useful to also point out some of the thirds that emerged. I think it is Benjamin's (2004) definition of the relational third that most captures the process between me and Marianne: "A quality or experience of intersubjective relatedness that has as its correlate a certain kind of mental space" (p. 7). This relational third refers to an innate sense of self with other that we bring to every meeting; it is the process by which we share experience with each other both consciously and unconsciously. It is within this cocreated space that one can directly access the other's emotional experience (Hargaden & Fenton, 2005). Although the relational third is the main context for the numinous moments described here, it will deepen appreciation of the depth of this encounter by recognizing other thirds, in particular, reflections on the cultural archetypal thirds evoked by the picture on the wall, the image of Hestia, the reveries on feminization connecting me with the internalizing subjugating father, the wind, and the wise old woman. All of these help us to capture something of the multiple metaphorical experiences of the clinical encounter.

Conclusion

Hestia was the most influential and widely revered of the Greek goddesses. Her name means *the essence,* that is, the true nature of things. It was through such transformative moments that Marianne was able to find her true nature. This eventually involved her making choices that led her to find joy in another relationship with a man, someone who both liked and respected her. Marianne was now conscious enough to cocreate a meaningful, satisfying life with a companion.

I realize that in the work I have described in this chapter, I departed almost totally from what would be recognized as classical transactional analysis. Yet the influence of my training in TA and the sense of classical transactional analysis as part of how I think, intuit, and assess is an integrated part of how I work. I value measurable outcomes, for instance, and hence the significance of measuring Marianne's change. It is important that there is a contract so that therapist and client know why and what they think they are doing in the room together, and Marianne and I continuously negotiated what we were doing and why. In many of my shared reflections with her, I used terms such as "Child ego state," "script," "games," and other transactional analysis terms. Over the years, though, my relational perspective has taken me beyond classical TA thinking toward incorporating the imaginative realm in the clinical encounter.

REFLECTIONS

The inspiration for this chapter came from my increasing consciousness of how the intersubjective process influences us. We are not in control of this influence, but having a third eye to the therapeutic couple reveals the unconscious in quite arbitrary and stunning ways, as described in the chapter. Marianne committed herself to the therapy and that was a wonderful gift for me, as the therapist, and for us as the therapeutic couple. I enjoyed so much of the work, traveling around the twists and turns of her mind forcing me to do the same. When I wrote the chapter, we thought Marianne had finally found herself. As it turned out, there were several years to go before she was finally freed to be the courageous, interesting, incredibly talented woman she is.

Chapter 3

"Father, Where Art Thou?" The Significance of Transgenerational Trauma in a Psychotherapy with Luke

Helena Hargaden

In this chapter, I begin with a short review of epigenetic theory (Yehuda et al., 2014; Yehuda et al., 2005) and propose a link with the transactional analysis concept of *episcript* intuitively described by Fanita English (1969). I introduce my client, Luke, describing the therapy contract and the progress and process of the therapy as it pertains to transgenerational trauma. I briefly outline the theory of the *domains of transference* (Hargaden & Sills, 2002) and show how I used this theory to guide me through the unfolding unconscious processes. I draw on the research by Rogers (2008) and her interpretations of Lacan to show how I was supported in my reflective process.

The Theory of Transgenerational Trauma: How the Past Informs the Present

The most recent research and a consequent paradigm shift in psychoanalysis/psychotherapy are arguably in the area of epigenetics, which involves a scientific study of transgenerational trauma. The nature of trauma means it has not been metabolized or mentalized (Fonagy & Target, 1998) but is often somatized. In the emerging theory of epigenetics, scientists have discovered that trauma is coded in the body in terms of cortisol levels and receptor site alterations (Yehuda et al., 2014). Research carried out on pregnant women involved in the World Trade Center attacks on September 11, 2001, in New York discovered low cortisol levels in the women and their newborn infants. In other research projects, Yehuda et al. (2014) proposed that transgenerational trauma is passed through the womb. They found that a traumatic trigger in the present often activates transgenerational trauma. These "ghosts" (unmetabolized trauma) remain in the embryo.

Although this research is in its infancy, it makes intuitive sense. For instance, English (1969) coined the phrase the episcript, using the metaphor of the "hot potato" to describe how a script can be passed down unconsciously through generations. It was an intuitive way of thinking that anticipated what is now reflected in the science of epigenetics. It is conceivable that those of us drawn to deeply examine our lives because of personal

DOI: 10.4324/9781032266237-4

suffering have perhaps found it incumbent on us to be the "chosen ones." By this, I refer to those of us who seem required, perhaps by our family constellation, to catch the hot potato, to be the ones who metabolize inherited transgenerational trauma.

Rogers (2008) captured the challenge for both therapist and client when she used the metaphor of trauma as an experience of *time stopping*; there is a deadened quality to it. In her case studies, Rogers used the Lacanian theory of *signifiers* (Lacan, 1977), which describe how words carry codes that, if examined, can point us in the direction of an underlying meaning. Trauma is, therefore, not available for change through cognitive methods alone but occupies a part of our psyche, often in the format of deadness, nothingness, and emptiness (Freud, 1917/1957; Green, 2005; Leader, 2008). When an experience of loss is avoided or repressed, it is unknown, so there can be no mourning. Instead, a melancholic fugue descends on the victim, keeping him or her from feeling truly alive (Freud, 1917/1957). Winnicott (1985) described the sublime beauty and purity of the maternal gaze, but what if the gaze that is reflected back to the infant is contaminated with brokenness and grief? What then is ingested and introjected with the mother's milk?

Mother, You Had Me, but I Never Had You (Lennon, 1970)

Luke was in his early 40s when he first came to see me. He had successfully dealt with specific behavioral concerns with a counselor and was a highly functioning professional holding a responsible position in his field of work. He came to me because he recognized that although he appeared to be confident on the outside, on the inside, it was a different story. He suffered from deep, and to him incomprehensible, insecurities that manifested in an inchoate sense of self. As we talked, it became clear to both of us that he had come to me to find his "self." When he told me the story of his childhood, he referred to moments of extreme brutality and extremes of physical and emotional neglect in a factual way, detached from any feeling. He told me that his mother had been an alcoholic and only became sober when Luke was about 6.

As his narrative unfolded, I began to recognize that when she became sober, Luke's mother had ruled her family like a cult. Her way of "mothering" had a strong flavor of subjugating narcissism (Shaw, 2014). Shaw described how the subjugating narcissist uses the power structure (in this instance, the power inherent in being the mother) to silence other subjectivities. Subjugating narcissists are usually intelligent and charismatic and use this to convince their group (in this case, the family) that only one subjectivity is valid, and in Luke's situation that was his mother's. When Luke described his childhood, it was his mother's story he told.

Luke's mother had been adopted. Her birth mother was a young woman, pregnant in the 1940s, but the story was vague. At one point, it seemed she might be Polish. Was she a Jewish immigrant fleeing persecution, we wondered? Or maybe she was a Catholic since she had been adopted into an Irish Catholic family. Who was Luke's birth father? Had his mother been raped? There were few facts, just suppositions. I was curious that Luke's mother did not seem interested in her own lineage or the meaning for her of being adopted. The only verifiable fact that emerged about Luke's grandmother was that after she had had her child adopted, she married and had six other children. Luke's mother also had six children. This seemed to be the only conscious sense of her attachment to her birth story as far as Luke understood it. Yet for a young girl in the 1940s to be pregnant, alone, and possibly without family would have been, at the least, a social catastrophe, something not to be talked about, a situation too shameful, making the woman vulnerable. Such a painful story, of course, put Luke's mother's behavior into context. It was perhaps the only way she knew or could conceive of to look after her family and keep a semblance of a functioning family.

When Luke talked about his mother, he often expressed extreme rage, the roots of which were most consciously caused by a conflict between his congruent felt sense of his subjectivity and his felt sense of a requirement that he accept his mother's narrative unquestioningly. Luke instinctively distrusted his mother in most things. For instance, he scorned her sudden conversion from Catholicism to Buddhism, which overnight turned the religious affiliation of the family from one set of beliefs to another. She did this without negotiation, discussion, or interest in how her children might feel or what they might want for themselves. As was her way, his mother used the family power structure to silence all other subjectivities. Throughout his life, Luke and his siblings had been emotionally steamrolled by their mother's personal trauma. This appeared to involve issues of sexual abuse and the Roman Catholic Church, which, as is well known, has received widespread global condemnation for the atrocities committed. Luke, however, had always instinctively (but secretly) questioned her narrative. As we talked through the actuality of his mother's experience (which had been written down in statements for her children to read and to sympathize with), it seemed that she had used a minor situation to ride the crest of an internationally renowned wave of censure against the Catholic Church. Together, Luke and I came to reflect that quite probably the underlying trauma—the loss of her birth mother, the circumstance in which she was conceived and later adopted—constituted a loss that remained hidden, unknown, and unmourned. It seemed likely that his mother unconsciously redefined her initial loss with a negative experience that she had in her childhood. She used this experience as her own cause célèbre by engaging in a battle with the Catholic Church. When I reflected on the type of emotional and psychological predicament, Luke felt himself to be in my reverie, took me to the haunting melody and lyrics of "Donna, Donna" by Zeitlin and Secunda (1941). In their song, written initially in Yidish, they describe the plight of the poor calves bound for slaughter and that if they wished to be free, they needed to learn to fly, like the swallow. In this metaphorical state, I knew that my work would be to to teach Luke how to fly like the swallow.

Father

The first time Luke mentioned his father, he told me that when he was seven years old, his father had left home. His five siblings were in tears, but Luke remembered that he only felt relieved, pretending to cry, he said, to hide his true feelings. In other references to his father, I came to think of him as a violent, alcoholic, demonic figure. Over the years we worked together, Luke repeated the story of his father leaving the home. It was like a mantra ("a sacred text used as an incantation; chanted or repeated inwardly in meditation," *Chambers Dictionary,* 2014, p. 931). Mantras induce an altered state of consciousness, and I now believe that Luke's repetitive referencing to the scene of his father's leaving the family, and his assertion that he was glad about it, induced a hypnotic hold over both of us. Father was bad. Good riddance to father. It has become clear to me that I picked up an unconscious prohibition that we were not to think about the father. On the periphery of my mind, I had some questions, but at that time, I was unable to access them so strong was the prohibition. Maybe, too, I was using the introjective domain to put on "hold" (Slochower, 1996) further questions, such as why was Luke the only one not to feel the loss of his father? What made the others cry? Were they fond of him? Was their father someone a child could feel fond of? More symbolically, another question began to form in my mind as the therapy progressed. Was Luke chosen unconsciously by his mother to experience her untold and unmourned history (as is discussed later here)? Were Luke's words describing an absence? Something that could not be talked about?

A Vengeful Mother Who Inflicts Wounds on Her Male Children

A recurring theme in Luke's story was his experience of abandonment by his mother. At age 14, he had been evicted from the family home for stealing money from his stepfather. At the age of 21, suffering from a near-fatal illness, his mother told him he could not return home for fear of contaminating his stepfather (a melodramatic overreaction). At a later stage in his adulthood, when Luke had a period of severe stress related to work and relationship pressures, she again was unable to offer comfort. Naturally, his sense of betrayal ran deep. Over my 30-odd years as a psychotherapist, I have often observed about myself and my clients that hidden in our childhood wounds, we can often find deep creativity and emotional strength. This was certainly true of Luke. From the beginning, he impressed me with his acuity and intuitive sense of things. As Luke witnessed his mother's coercive ways—such as the multiple contradictions in her unreciprocal demands for loyalty and love—he developed a finely tuned radar for the "truth" of a situation. He learned to pick up on inconsistencies quickly. His creative intuitive temperament probably saved him from the fate of his three brothers: One died tragically young, one developed severe mental health problems, and the third presents an impenetrable macho face to the world.

Given this history, I was surprised and confused by Luke's protective behavior toward his mother. He often offered her useful advice and in the past had loaned her large sums of money. I began to think about Luke's symbiosis with his mother as a type of folie à deux that would go some way to explain why he still experienced his power and self-knowledge as potentially dangerous and catastrophic.

Understandably, the therapy with Luke involved intense relational projections between us, with my honesty, truth, and subjectivity coming under intense scrutiny. Our work required me to reflect on my internal self-states, their potential meanings, and the use of my own transgenerational trauma to deepen my understanding of what might be at stake for Luke when trying to find his "self." We traversed turbulent times together. During this process, I found it theoretically supportive to think about the domains of transference (Hargaden & Sills, 2002) as a way to chart the complex dynamics that existed between us. Here I want to briefly outline the theory of the domains of transference as a prelude to demonstrating how the transferential processes emerged in differing forms throughout the therapy with Luke.

The Domains of Transference

The domains of transference (Hargaden & Sills, 2002) are based on the idea that transference is ubiquitous and brings the therapist and client into a relational process that can be examined through three different, coexisting theoretical lenses. When creating this model, Charlotte Sills and I benefited from working in the fertile atmosphere of theoretical pluralism created at the Metanoia Institute by its founding member Petruska Clarkson. Moiso (1985), Clarkson (1991), and Moiso and Novellino (2000) were the major transactional analysts who reflected our clinical and training experiences most accurately. Retrospectively, I believe that our feminism, based on the challenge to patriarchal attitudes (seeing women as objects), was also significant in our search for theoretical perspectives that allowed for a subject-subject connection described by Stark (2000) as a *two-person psychotherapy*. For more detailed references to the sources of the domains of transference, see Hargaden and Sills (2002), where we acknowledge, in depth, all of our sources.

The three domains are briefly described as follows. The *introjective transference* involves the developmental needs of clients that have never been met, such as mirroring and validation of internal feeling states to support the development of a healthy narcissistic sense of self (Kohut, 1971). The *projective transference* involves the splitting and projection (Klein, 1975/1988; Moiso & Novellino, 2000) that occurs when a person is overwhelmed by feelings and experiences that have never been expressed and made meaning of through metabolization with a reflective other. The *transformational transference* refers to primitive affective experiences that are encoded in the psyche, have never come into consciousness, and are linked to traumatic phenomena that can only find meaning through a process of *projective identification* (Klein, 1975/1988). Projective identification means that the client invokes feelings in the therapist as a way of conveying the person's unconscious, unmetabolized feelings and experience and requires the therapist to do something about them. As Bollas (1987) put it, "In order to find the patient we must look for him within ourselves" (p. 202). In the traditional psychoanalytic view of projective identification, the analyst is required to make a transference interpretation based on the idea that the client is projecting an alien feeling into the analyst. From a humanistic perspective, the therapist is expected to think of the feeling as only pertaining to her or his psyche/pathology. Sills and I (Hargaden & Sills, 2002) argued that if the therapist is experiencing a feeling, no matter how odd it seems, it belongs to her or him and to the relationship with the client. The therapist is, therefore, required to examine it from the perspective of mutuality and the bidirectionality of the relational unconscious. The next step is to look for the meaning of her or his feelings, to be willing, in the process, to be changed, and to use those introspective reflections as a way to deepen the meaning of what is happening in the therapeutic relationship. Thus, the term "transformational" pertains to both therapist and client: Both will be changed.

The Transferential Domains as They Emerged in the Therapy with Luke

"The more insecure and ruptured the earlier attachments were, the more fragile the sense of self will be and some patients will implicate the therapist in a multi-transferential relationship" (Hargaden & Sills, 2002, p. 50). Throughout my work with Luke, all transferential domains coexisted, varying in intensity and degree depending on what the focus of the work was. From the beginning, I felt a strong sense of Luke's developmental needs, not only from the perspective of the concrete information about his earliest experiences but from my feelings of protectiveness toward him as I attuned to his archaic Child ego states. When I examined my feelings, it made sense to link them to his maternal deprivation. My initial countertransferential response was, therefore, clearly linked to the introjective transference. For instance, as I worked by keeping on the trail of Luke's altering mind, I became a congruent witness to his experiences. I validated and mirrored his internal "witness," who had observed inconsistencies throughout his childhood. This transferential process enabled Luke to gradually introject his relational experience of my attuned mirroring and thus begin to engage empathically with his vulnerable self-states. This process is understood as the development of healthy narcissism (Kohut, 1971) and enables the client to experience "an evolving sense of his 'self'" (Hargaden & Sills, 2002, p. 52).

However, as comfortable as this process often feels because it is soothing and harmonious, it is unsustainable if psychic change is to happen. From this perspective, it was fortunate that Luke was also in group therapy with me. The therapy group is made up of psychotherapists only. There is often a reflective process, and at times this evoked in Luke the projective transference. From his experience of me as "ideal" in the individual therapy setting, he found it more difficult in the group situation where his terror and mistrust of closeness were highlighted. His alert mind was wired to notice any inconsistency, any intuitive sense he had of my incongruence. When he had a feeling that I might be telling him what to think or how to behave, he felt betrayed, that he had lost the "good" me and was back on his own again, feeling himself to be subjugated and therefore alerting him to the prospect of being abandoned unless he "towed the line." It was helpful at these time to return to the individual setting where, together, we could make meaning of his sense of loss, fear of abandonment, and rage about the subjugating attitudes that he had experienced with his mother, father, and some of his siblings. As we conversed/struggled together, he began to integrate both the "good" and "bad" parts of me, and then I became a more stable object, neither all good nor all bad.

The Transformational Transference and Transgenerational Trauma

It is in this transferential domain that the unconscious legacies of trangenerational trauma will most reveal themselves. Projective identification sneaks into one's system like a psychological snake, taking over one's mind and heart in ways that require a good deal of reflection. Certainly this was my experience with Luke. On many occasions, I experienced feeling penetrated by feelings and thoughts that on the surface were not immediately recognizable as mine. On the surface, the sessions were often explicit and interpersonal, but under the noise of these exchanges I often came away conscious of many other sounds that required my attention. Through my dreams, reflections, introspection, and self-analysis, I discovered more nuanced ways to think as I reflected on my feelings of anxiety and a sense that a feeling of rage and desperation could not be soothed. I found these feelings intolerable and difficult to own. In this sense, much of the therapeutic work was done outside of the sessions, probably by both of us. As Mitchell (1997) wrote, "Good analytic technique concerns not correct actions but hard thinking, in a continual process of reflection and consideration" (p. 268). I describe further the background to some of the feelings that emerged for me.

The Background to the Therapist's Subjectivity

A few years previous to my work with Luke, I became interested in trans-generational trauma after attending the 2013 Wounds of History Conference in New York hosted by the International Association of Relational Psychoanalysts. The conference generated a great deal of research about unmetabolized transgenerational trauma from Jewish and African American scholars in relation to the Holocaust and African American legacies of slavery. Although specific to those groups of people, the research demonstrated the ubiquity of transgenerational trauma. Coming from an Irish background, I experienced the conference as a validation and witness of my inherited transgenerational trauma. I realized that the novel I had been writing was my way of continuing to try to metabolize the trauma buried in my Irish background.

As the therapy with Luke progressed, I found myself reflecting *yet again* on my own disturbed transgenerational trauma, which involved intense betrayals, experiences of not belonging, splitting, and repression of painful wounds. Initially, I wanted to disavow the feelings and experiences that were emerging for me. I told myself that I had *already done this work.* I was reminded, however, by this process that no matter how much work we do on ourselves in our own therapy, we cannot change the past. When there is intense trauma in our background, we can only alleviate the pain by becoming conscious and by searching for its meaning (Frankl, 1946/1959).

Over a period of several months, I found myself reflecting on my own transgenerational trauma. The question I asked myself was, why now? Was it connected to the therapy with Luke? There were several triggers. One was on a difficult trip I made to Ireland just after a session with Luke in which he had expressed despair that I was just not getting his sense of betrayal alongside his fear of it. After a painful conversation with my cousin in which I felt betrayed by her, something I would normally have shrugged off, putting it down to her oft-expressed generalized anger, I made links between what was happening between me and my cousin and our shared traumatic ancestral Irish history. I had various disturbing dreams, and, fortunately, I still had an opportunity to make further meaning in my own analysis as once again I touched on the wounds inherent in my history. I believe the deeply subjective process I found myself in was linked to an unconscious experience with Luke, that he wanted me to make meaning of something about him that I seemed incapable of doing. Or, perhaps more significantly, it was something I could not feel with him until I had allowed myself to feel as he had—betrayed—as we shall see later in this narrative.

My Transgenerational Trauma

I have always had a conscious understanding of the extremes of trauma suffered by the Irish, such as the famines of the 19th century, which reduced the population by 25%. There was also the complex subject of centuries of British colonization, which culminated in the Irish Uprising of 1916 and led to a bloody civil war that caused massive upheaval in Ireland. As I thought about these things again, I wondered if the worst trauma for the Irish, and certainly one that formed a consciously negative influence on my own psyche, was the rigid nationalist rule of De Valera from 1959–1973. Together with the Irish Catholic Church, he exerted a tyrannous, misogynistic, and puritanical rule, during which time it has now emerged, many thousands of children were sexually abused under the auspices of the church, and the whole population was severely restricted in how they lived their lives.

My Personal History

The background of my Irish family is full of betrayals, losses, and intolerable truths. My grandfather, a member of the Royal Irish Constabulary until the 1916 Uprising, was overnight identified as "a traitor to the cause" because he had been in the pay of the British government (which all such professionals were before the Republic was formed). His wife, my grandmother, on the other hand, had been engaged to a rebel fighter in 1916 who had died in the Uprising. My grandparents met and married from opposite sides of the unrest, and in doing so, paradoxically, both lost their sense of belonging. Although the Uprising afforded me the possibility of being born since my grandmother's first fiancé died on the battlefield, it left a legacy of not belonging (Hargaden & Tudor, 2016), of being cast out of the community like the proverbial scapegoat.

All of these events have affected/infected my family constellation. Prior to my own psychotherapy, I carried a fearless sense of defiance, intolerable sorrow, and the despair of victimhood, which could not be explained alone by my childhood experience. In her groundbreaking book on the subject of madness and transgenerational trauma, Rogers (2008) argued that to listen to just the "victim" erases subjectivity, morality, choice, complexity, and the capacity to transform suffering into strength. This poses a challenge to us all as both clients and psychotherapists. Naturally, as psychotherapists, we have to find a way to validate and witness traumatic legacies yet steer away from staying with the victimhood of them. It is, therefore, crucially important for therapists to work through their own traumatic inheritance. Otherwise, there will be a temptation to stay with the victimhood of the traumatized person, relying on empathic understanding alone as a vehicle for therapeutic change. Unconscious traumatic legacies often lie at the heart of unspoken and unknown anxieties, terrors, and sorrows. Learning to live more consciously with what we are born with enables therapists to think more clinically about the significance of clients' past histories. From this perspective, therapists can act as genuine witnesses to the suffering because they can use their own transgenerational lens to focus on the multiplicity of unconscious forms that emerge in therapy.

Why the Therapist's Subjective Experience?

When working with transgenerational trauma, we are looking for something that cannot be said or represented (Rogers, 2008). Understanding this put Luke's "mantra" about his "lack of feelings" for his father into perspective. He was trying to tell me something that I initially failed to decode. Clients depend on their therapist tuning in to what has not been represented and is therefore not known so they can hear themselves through the experience of the therapist (Lacan, 1977). The clinical effect of owning and reflecting on my historical legacy ever more consciously enabled me to become deeply attuned to Luke.

Symbols Leading to the Past

From this perspective, I began to wonder if some of the feelings triggered in the therapy with Luke reflected his mother's intolerable experience, which may have been passed on to Luke unconsciously because he was the most responsive to her needs (as described earlier). I wondered if Luke's unmet needs might mirror his mother's unmet needs and how he had perhaps introjected her needs. For example, he remembered that his mother had once referred to being sold to her adoptive family. I thought this symbolic of an unbearable truth. I wondered how the meaning of this disturbing thought had underpinned the unconscious family dynamic. As Luke's recall of what he knew became stronger, he realized that it was only his mother who was an alcoholic, not his father.

This information made it more possible to refer to Luke's father and at the same time to express curiosity about his continued lack of interest in knowing about him. Luke was mostly disinterested in the subject, and when he did have a conversation with me about his father, I wondered if he was acquiescing to my need to know rather than his own. Or maybe my hopefulness was experienced as an unconscious unwillingness to bear witness to the psychic annihilation he had experienced from his mother (Shaw, 2014).

On the other hand, Luke's apparent disinterest may have been because he did not have a conscious way of knowing the answer to the question. A breakthrough came when Luke's partner discovered Luke's father on Facebook. From this chance "encounter," Luke learned that his father, far from being the demon he had always been described as, seemed to have led a constructive life. He appeared to be living happily with a new partner and her family and was particularly interested in the natural world. This stirred some interest in Luke, and we discussed how he might contact his father. He wrote a letter for me to read, but he did not show it to me and it was never posted. The subject of his father died a death, again. Shortly after this episode, I commented on his difficulty in thinking about contacting his father. This time we got closer to the root of the matter: "Helena, you don't understand." Luke leaned forward in his chair. His body language seemed to be imploring me to comprehend something for which he had no words. Eventually, he exclaimed, "It's in my DNA, Helena. It is in my DNA. I can't betray my mother."

I felt shocked. My body became rigid. He seemed to be telling me that we had come to the end of the line. Maybe his father could not stay alive in the therapy. Was Luke transferring into me what had been unconsciously projected into him? I connected my bodily reaction with the movement Luke had made, that in leaning forward, he was acting out a thrusting movement that I received as a type of penetration. During these brief moments, I thought about his grandmother, who had been impregnated, not by a husband or a named man. She would, of course, have been shocked. I thought about his mother carrying a birth trauma of no named father and then sold for money. In those moments, Luke conveyed a sense of his terror and fear of not only betrayal but being a betrayer. He was essentially describing the cellular level of his experience. So strong was my experience that I took it to my analyst, who thought it had the hallmarks of an oedipal process. Had Luke become enmeshed in the trauma of his mother's experience? Maybe even the generation before her? There can be no certainty here. Did he want to kill his father because he wanted his mother for himself? Had be been appropriated by his mother to metaphorically kill his father and stay enmeshed with his mother, symbolized by the concept of the DNA? I describe next how together we navigated these thoughts.

It is through these types of reflections that I realized that there were major themes of betrayal, terror, and shame of being cast out, as my grandfather had been for not being on the "right" side after the Uprising. My poor grandmother, too, found herself on the "wrong" side when she had always fought to be a true Fenian and therefore on the "right" side of the Uprising. Then, through marriage, she was on the "wrong" side. I think about how Luke wanted me to recognize something of the demonic spirit contained in his reference to his DNA and the terror of betrayal that lurked underneath. A question began to formulate: Are we to be loyal to our family, a belief, or an ideology at the expense of being loyal to ourselves? My history and reflections on my personal background required me to keep different perspectives in the frame when working with Luke. I was now more consciously sensitive to Luke's terror of betraying his mother and of being betrayed. His mother had once been betrayed, abandoned as an infant, and also we can presume her mother was betrayed by the man who made her pregnant. All of this was only a hypothesis, and yet it felt right. It was through the transformational transferential process that Luke pushed his unconscious into mine so he could find who he is, so that I could work at decoding what was being pushed into me and make it relevant for his life. Clearly, it was not necessary for me to self-disclose. Instead, I needed to reflect, think, and analyze my subjectivity so I could find a way to further the therapeutic process. If Luke was to fly, like the swallow, I had to find him in my unconscious, and to do that I had to reexamine my own transgenerational trauma. Only then could I feel why the terror of betrayal and the dreadful consequences of it was a major theme in Luke's story, his mother's story, and quite possibly beyond.

Luke

Luke demanded that I understand that what I was asking of him was impossible. "It is in my DNA!" Although it is understood that the emotional transmission of trauma is through attachment (Bowlby, 1958), this did not help us find a way through the impasse in which we found ourselves. Something was off limits and out of reach of reflective thought. "Trauma is so much like tipping a globe and watching the snow descend on the same scene in the same way. Whatever is unresolved and unsayable repeats" (Rogers, 2008, p. 97). The snow had descended on us, on the therapy. I even began to think, well, maybe Luke's father does not really matter after all. There lingered between Luke and me unconscious phantasies of punishment. Somehow, Luke's witnessing—and my witnessing of him—felt dangerous. Destruction was in the air. Meaning making was threatened with destruction.

Luke—and Theory Matters

Shortly after the DNA episode in the work with Luke, I enrolled in a colloquium on transgenerational trauma. It was there that I learned more about the emerging theory of epigenetics as described earlier. I learned that epigenetics is the theory of transgenerational trauma. I knew then that the best way through to Luke was to appeal to his intelligence, his ability to reflect, and his natural curiosity. So, I brought the subject of epigenetics into our discussion to shed light on the mysteries of experience and unfelt knowns. Unexpectedly, we concluded that if molecules are involved, there was nothing to be ashamed or frightened of in the here and now. I shared some of my findings from the research described earlier (Yehuda et al., 2014; Yehuda et al., 2005), making links with Luke's comment about DNA. Luke's use of "DNA" suggested that his fear of betraying his mother was at a cellular level of his experience.

It was the sixth year of therapy with Luke, who in the meantime had trained and qualified as a psychotherapist. There was a strong bond of trust between us, and we were able to talk about many things and possibilities, to play with different interpretations, and to allow for dissonance between us. I know I must be patient. In research for this article, I reread Annie Rogers's *The Unsayable* and was reminded of the "lack" in mother that the child attempts to fill with a "phallus" (Lacan, 1977). By this, I understood Lacan to propose that all children will pick up an experience of something missing in their mother. The phallus symbolizes something to compensate for that shortcoming. The more sensitively attuned child, and maybe the one co-opted, will attempt to fill this lack in the mother. I shared these thoughts with Luke. We played with the idea that Luke was the "chosen one": chosen to fill a hole in his mother and maybe also to cure his grandmother, who had been a teenager, possibly violated by a man and thus requiring a man who could make her better, although Luke never could.

"It's in My DNA, Helena—I Can't Betray My Mother."

These interpretative sessions altered something in Luke and between us. Luke began coming into therapy feeling "blank," which was quite unusual. His blankness proved to be a rich source of emergent feelings and reflections. It was in this process that Luke recovered memories of happier times in his childhood: time spent in loving companionship with his mother, eating banana sandwiches and watching his favorite cartoons. It struck me that this maybe was a time when their bond was "sealed."

I wrote the first draft of this chapter so far during a two-week break. As is well known in our profession, our minds are connected at levels that we do not fully understand. This is what happened after the break.

After the Break

"I wrote a letter to my father," Luke told me by way of greeting. He went on to say that his mother had discovered his father's details on Facebook. Luke did not tell her he already knew. He felt this might get in the way of contacting his father and was worried that the whole family would become involved. I said, "Yes. Maybe you need to make a preemptive strike."

Luke told me that ten minutes prior to the session, his mother texted him to tell him she loved him. He was shocked. I was shocked. His mother knew nothing about his therapy and therefore his session times, and she never used that type of language. We mulled this over together. I read his letter. It was quite anodyne, and after a while, I read it again and asked him if he would like to see his father. Yes, was his definite answer. So I said, why not ask that directly in the letter? He went off to revise and then post his letter.

By our next session, his father had not replied, and Luke was full of feelings he had never known in relation to him: sadness, sorrow, longing, desire, and fear. I felt anxious too but hopeful. By our next session, his father had replied. He had received Luke's letter as he was turning the key in his home for the last time. He was moving to another house. The "pre-emptive strike" came to my mind! The letter was measured in tone but warm, inviting, and respectful. Luke and I both shed some tears.

We have been (and still are) on a relational journey together with no certain destination in mind but with much disturbance and emotional upheaval for both of us. He, me, we are in a transformative process. Luke will see his father. He is writing him a long letter. We have arrived some-where. Luke tells me he feels changed, and it is in his body. He feels he has more oxygen to breathe, that he has been powering on through life mis-aligned, and that the left side of his body has been released as he owns the right-hand side of his body. "I can't say more—I just feel lighter. I can breathe." We think this has more to do with separating from his mother than finding his father. Maybe it is both! I think of the song cited at the beginning of this chapter. Maybe Luke is finding his wings like the swallow, learning to fly. The swallow is also a symbol of the soul. Is Luke's visceral sense of feeling liberated a release of his soul? I looked up the meaning of the name Luke (not his real name), curious as to why I used chosen it as a pseudonym. In biblical terms, it means the "bringer of light." This feels meaningful to me because this is what has happened through this process: The light has shone on the therapy and on us both.

In Summary

Naturally, the way of working described in this article poses challenging, uncomfortable questions about the line between attunement/resonance with a client and collusion/projective identifications. How can we think about this clinically? For me—and there will be more questions to pose and ways to think about this—two areas require attention. One is personal and the other is methodological. From the personal perspective, the therapist must dedi-cate herself or himself to self-examination with a qualified other. In my case, that has been with a Jungian analyst who works from a solid ethical frame of reference combining his psychotherapy approach with his vocation as a rabbi. From a methodological point of view, the theory of mentalization (Fonagy & Target, 1998) provides a way of thinking that opens a more neutral psychological space between therapist and client in which the client is required to analyze the therapist's words and make his or her own meaning out of them. (For a more detailed critique of relational transac-tional analysis, see Cornell & Hargaden, 2020).

In this chapter, I have offered a way to think about how transgenerational trauma can affect some aspect of the development of the mind. As described, the therapeutic process involved both therapist and client in complex rela-tional transferential processes and required a willingness on the part of both to stay in conflictual intensity, confusion, and the uncertainty of a hazardous psychological journey. The crucial learning from this experience, as demonstrated in this chapter, is the significance of transgenerational trauma as a hidden process that has never been represented.

It is my foundational training in classical transactional analysis that provides me with a theoretical container in which I ask myself: Is this therapy working? What are the measurable outcomes? In the therapy described here, Luke changed. He has become the author of his own life, has taken full responsibility for himself, and has moved on from his rage with his mother. What is his measurement of the therapy we have done? Today, when writing my final draft of this chapter, I asked Luke what he had made of my self-disclosures in the article. He said that he read them as a biography. I persisted, "Yes, but how did it feel to read about my 'stuff'?" "It made sense," he said. "It made me feel interconnected with you. It made me know, with certainty, that I had been on your mind."

REFLECTIONS

My reflections are brief for this chapter because so many of my meditative thoughts are contained therein. By the time I worked with Luke, I was able to understand how the client moves into the therapist's mind and that this requires significant reflective capacity in the therapist. In this chapter, I link traumatizing narcissism to family cults and make a link with how transgenerational trauma infects the family system. I had been greatly influenced by my work with Maya Wallfisch and the Wounds of History conference I attended in New York 2013. I learned that transgenerational trauma is ubiquitous and that the main psychological problem is that something extremely traumatic has not been witnessed. Descendants are subject to the parents trauma. They travel through a world which is experienced as the dead third. My research into the literature formed an essential part of this case. As can be seen from the chapter, I was involved in deeply personal experiences which I synthesized with the case studies and theoretical perspectives that emerged from this conference to help me find meaning for myself and my client. I have rarely worked with someone who seemed to propel me on my own journey so painfully, so that I could participate in this journey, even though the content of our histories were different. Luke was extremely psychological, sensitive, musical; so together we made music—only some of which required translation! It was an incredible psychotherapy in so many ways, one of which was unless the client wants to "go there," there is nothing much the therapist can do! It is a two-way street. I am deeply grateful to Luke and his adamantine, courageous determination, and ability to work through his trauma.

Chapter 4

Deconfusion of the Child Ego State

A Relational Perspective

Helena Hargaden and Charlotte Sills

Eric Berne (1961/1986) implied that deconfusion was an integral part of structural analysis: "Psychoanalytic cure in structural terms means deconfusion of the Child with a largely decontaminated Adult as a therapeutic ally" (p. 162). However, he also revealed an ambivalent attitude toward working with the dynamic Child, sometimes referring rather dismissively to the "luxury" (p. 149) of analyzing the Child and other times suggesting deconfusion as a phase of treatment.

In our clinical work, we have noticed an increase in the prevalence of patients who present with symptoms that require resolution within the Child ego state (as noted by Clark, 1991), especially those who manifest schizoid processes. It has, therefore, been increasingly necessary to pay attention to the phase of treatment known as deconfusion of the Child ego state.

There is already a distinguished body of work in the transactional analysis literature that considers deconfusion work (Blackstone, 1993; Clark, 1991; Erskine, 1991, 1993, 1994; Erskine & Trautmann, 1996; Haykin, 1980; Moiso, 1985; Shmukler, 1991). We seek to build on this tradition by expanding transactional analysis theory to incorporate a theory of self that is useful in mapping the complex processes involved in the deconfusion phase of treatment. Using our theory of self in the Child ego state, we have integrated into transactional analysis some principles from object relations and self psychology, theories that also focus on a notion of the self. In doing so, we have enriched our understanding of primary processes and complex mental states, while remaining within the transactional analysis model. We suggest that the transferential relationship is the vehicle for deconfusion and that the work is facilitated by a detailed analysis of this relationship.

Structural Analysis and Deconfusion

In proposing our theory of self, we recognize that our thinking is, of course, simply a story. We find it useful, however, for making sense of some of the complex processes involved in psychotherapy of the Child ego state. We

DOI: 10.4324/9781032266237-5

propose that C_2 is the whole "self" and that the internal organization of the "self" comprises C_1, A_1, and P_1. We link the internal organization of the self in C_2 with Stern's (1985) domains of the self. This is to underline the dynamic, constantly evolving, interactive nature of the internal relational world as symbolized by P_1, A_1, and C_1 (P_o/C_o).

C_1: The Core Self

We suggest that C_1 contains C_o and P_o (Sills, 1995). From this perspective, we understand C_o to be the emergent self (Stern, 1985) wherein the baby A is thought to occupy some kind of presocial, precognitive, preorganized life "phase" (p. 37). C_o is experienced as bodilyaffective states that include the sense of being contacted by the environment (mother), the latter of whom is represented in Figure 4.1 as P_o. C_o is the seat of the child's mirroring and idealizing yearnings. This constellation hints at the fragile yet dynamic nature of very early primitive processes, which are not accessible to memory but may only be uncovered through phenomenological inquiry based on careful attention to transferential phenomenon. The infant's experience of the mutual interaction with a selfregulating other (Stern, 1985) becomes, in our view, an integral part of the child's sense of a cohesive OK self, which we visualize as being contained in a type of amniotic sac of the A_o created by C_o/P_o (see Figure 4.1).

The purpose of the selfregulating mother/other is to enable the child to manage his feelings and experiences and remain feeling OK. When the mother is "good enough" (Winnicott, 1960), this task is completed in a way that enables the infant to integrate his experiences sufficiently to be able to tolerate his most primitive feelings and to instinctively develop selfesteem and appropriate grandiosity. The cohesive self grows from the interplay between the child's potential and the parents' selective responses. When there are sufficient experiences of attuned interplay between the child and the environment, he develops internalized representations of self and mother (C_o/P_o) to support the healthy development of a core self (A_o). However,

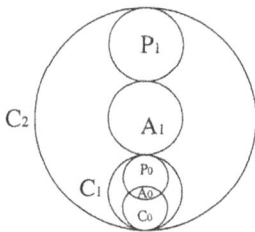

Figure 4.1 The Self: The Child Ego State.

when the infant experiences cumulative misattunement and nonattunement from the environment, he has no way of dealing with this except by splitting off the Aundigested" experiences (Klein, 1986). This can be understood as the schizoid process.

The Child, therefore, remains in a sense incomplete and unintegrated (A_o) despite the fact that she may have a coherent and consistent, though limited, sense of self. The splitoff, unintegrated experiences are walled inside C_o or form P_1 (Figure 4.2) along with the internalized the internalized representations of the other (described by Goulding and Goulding [1979] as injunctions). In this view of child development, it seems to us that C_1 is the foundation on which the rest of the self—A_1 and P_1—is built.

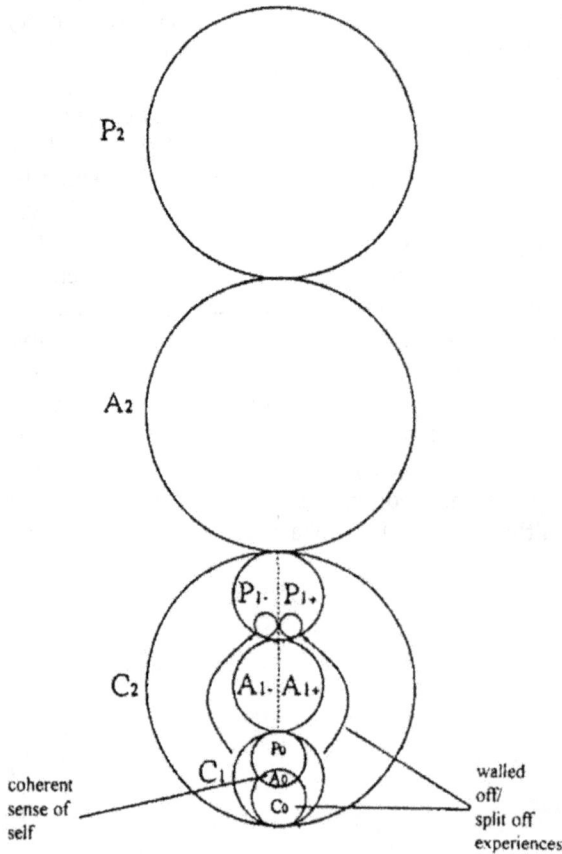

Figure 4.2 The Development of the Self.

A_1: The Verbal and Intersubjective Self

A_1 represents the child's attempts to make sense of self, others, and the world based on C_1 experiences and the subsequent patterns of his relationships. It is the foundation of the personality and has two faces: A_{1+} and A_{1-}. A_{1+} is the "I'm OK if I ..." and consists of the child's successful adaptations to the parents' counterscript messages. A_{1-} is the child's making sense of those moments of feeling that he has fallen from grace. He feels notOK and experiences negative injunctions. If the infant's needs are adequately met and his fundamental sense of OKness is intact, these two sides are reasonably successfully integrated and the child feels OK about himself and his activities.

For example, John learned that he could please his parents in many ways. As a baby he was loved and cherished, and this experience formed the basis of an OK sense of self (C_1). When he was a toddler, his parents approved of his curiosity and intelligence, received his love with joy, and were particularly gratified when he showed thoughtful caring for his baby brother. His sense of falling from grace, of notOKness, occurred when they reacted not only with disapproval but also with shock at his expression of jealous rage toward the loved brother or when he was rough and competitive with friends. He felt shame (A_{1-}) and at these moments connected with primitive shame (C_1). However, his parents knew how to reach out to him again, to forgive him and repair the rupture between them, so his shame never became unbearable. He was able to accept and integrate both A_{1+} and A_{1-} into his sense of self (Figure 4.3a).

In contrast, when the infant's relational needs are not adequately met, the child compensates by clinging to the positive image of herself (A_{1+}) and excluding the unmanaged, unaccepted feeling (C_1). She may develop an exaggerated sense of her own worth, or, paradoxically, an exaggerated humility, often accompanied by a sense of omnipotence (A_{1+}).

For example, Mary's alcoholic mother was alternately abusing and neglecting. Mary quickly shut down not only any grief, fear, and rage that she might have experienced but also her needs for love and prizing. The only positive attention she received was from her father, who was mainly absent but praised her for caring for her mother on those occasions when he was home. The defensive selfimage Mary created was of the flawless angel who selflessly cared for others and catered to their needs. She trained as a nurse, married, and was the perfect wife and mother. She anticipated every need of her friends and family, controlling them all with her love and care while simultaneously discounting her own needs and position. This inflated sense of worth/humility was designed to disguise her deep sense of worthlessness (A_{1-} and C_1).

Such script decisions in A_1 are born out of and built on the infant's experience (C_1) and therefore cannot truly be changed without prior or

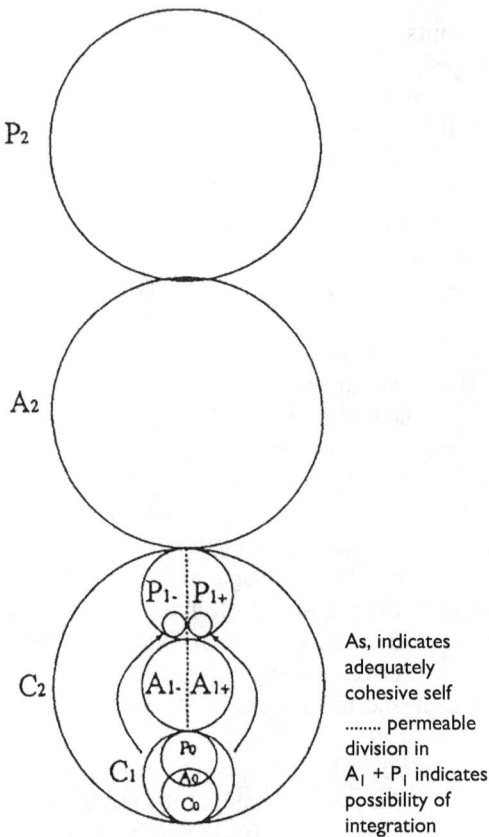

P₂

A₂

P₁₋ P₁₊

A₁₋ A₁₊

C₂

Po

C₁

Ao

Co

As, indicates
adequately
cohesive self

.... permeable
division in
$A_1 + P_1$ indicates
possibility of
integration

Figure 4.3a The Cohesive Self.

simultaneous change in the early bodily affective processes (C_1). For instance, if anyone complained of being controlled, or if Mary was found to be inadequate, she lost her sense of OKness. In this place (A_{1-}) she experienced again the rejecting and abusive mothering in the form of injunctions such as Don't Exist, Don't Be You, and Don't Look After Your Needs (P_{1-}). We would understand these processes as Mary's racket system.

When experiencing these feelings, Mary could be heard to complain that no one appreciated or understood her and that her needs were not important. We hypothesize that the psychological purpose of Mary's ongoing expressions of discontent were to keep her from experiencing the emptiness and despair in the core repressed (C_1) part of herself. While Mary's racket feelings may have been available for cognitive change, unless attention was paid to the underlying grief and desolation, significant aspects of her personality would remain walled off and isolated from contact.

Clearly, the greater the extent of the parenting deficit (and this could include intrusive parenting), the greater will be the split within A_1 and the more excluded will be C_1. Figure 4.3a shows a relatively cohesive self in A_o and a permeable division line in A_1 and P_1. Figure 4.3b demonstrates someone with more damage to the self. This is indicated by an "empty" self in C_1 and an impermeable split in A_1 and P_1. Since few people have ideal parenting, most have an element of this defensive organization. Individuals who are permanently depressed, anxious, and so on are stuck in A_{1-}, only too painfully aware of feelings of worthlessness. Part of the therapeutic task is to develop healthy narcissism, that is, A_{1+} built on a sense of selfesteem developed in C_1.

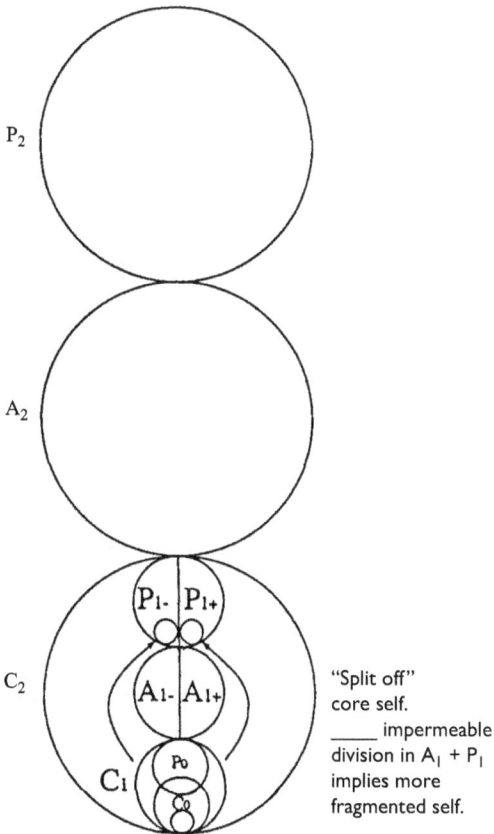

"Split off"
core self.

_____ impermeable
division in $A_1 + P_1$
implies more
fragmented self.

Figure 4.3b The Undeveloped Self.

P_1: The Internal Object Representation

P_1 comprises P_{1+} and P_{1-}. When the infant has experienced gross mis-attunement from the environment, she is unable to make sense of what is going on inside. For instance, when the child projects anxiety outward, she needs the environment to soothe and make sense of her experience. All those feelings that have not been adequately processed, including primary unscreened introjections, are intolerable to the infant, and to manage them, she makes them a part of self but splits off from them (pushing them into P_1). This intrapsychic process enables the infant to manage feelings that otherwise would threaten to overwhelm her. We find it useful, therefore, to think of P_1 as containing both introjects and denied parts of the natural self. In the example of Mary, her P_{1-} contains the injunctions from her mother (Don't Exist, Don't Be You, Don't Be Close,) and her own rejected hostile responses to her abusing mother. However, Mary managed to split off her P_{1-} most of the time, only falling prey to vicious selfhatred when the A_{1+} image failed. Her P_{1+}, however, contained a selfconstructed, idealized "other" who appreciated and admired her virtues. It contained elements of her father's adoration but was fleshed out by her own grandiose defense. P_1, therefore, contains both introjected images of the other and also elements of the self that have been rejected or created.

In this model, when the child has had a healthy enough childhood, the internal organization of C_2 comprises all these elements in a way that permits the person to grow and develop with a cohesive sense of self. In such cases, the Child, while certainly being limited by the imperfections of parenting and environment, contains a solid sense of core self.

In contrast, in our practice, we are seeing more people with disorders of the self ranging from mild to the more fractured sense of self seen in a personality disorder. When the internal organization of the Child ego state is fragile, integration can only take place within a relationship in which the therapist is willing to take part in the different psychological positions required of him or her. Such a need arises from the internal object world of the infant and materializes within the transferential relationship. Deconfusion, therefore, requires that the therapist be emotionally available and open to letting the relationship impact him or her.

When defined within the transferential relationship, the therapist's task in deconfusion is twofold. First, the therapist must be available for the impact of the patient's unintegrated experiences and projection, to help make sense of the material, and to enable the patient to integrate the splitoff parts. Second, he or she must pick up the unmet relational needs transferred from the Child and respond appropriately within the relationship. Both of these tasks of deconfusion involve a willingness on behalf of the therapist to engage himself or herself in affective processes while retaining an observing, objective Adult ego (see our later discussion about transference and countertransference).

To achieve deconfusion, the therapist needs to incorporate four inter-related steps, which form the treatment plan. Although these steps are neither linear nor meant as a definitive description, they are presented here in what we believe is the most logical order.

Step One: Development of the Empathic Relationship

The Empathic Transaction: "An empathic transaction occurs when the therapist communicates … understanding of what the patient is experiencing and the patient experiences being understood" (Clark, 1991, p. 93). We see this process initially (Figure 4.4) as a series of complementary transactions between the patient's Adult and the therapist and complementary ulterior transactions between the patient's Child and the therapist's Adult. "This is a necessary but not the sole condition for a 'good relationship'" (Berne, 1966/1994, p. 225). The therapist, therefore, needs to think about how to keep the transactions complementary in order to establish an empathic bond between patient and therapist.

For example, a patient may be saying that she is angry although the therapist senses sadness. If the patient experiences her sadness as anger, she needs to feel heard at this Aracket" level of communication before she will feel safe enough to go deeper. Thus, it is important initially to respond to the patient's felt meaning; although ultimately the therapist's task may be decontamination, she must respond with empathy and respect to the patient's contaminated Adult (Figure 4.5).

Eventually the empathic bond makes it possible for the patient to feel secure enough to revive unmet needs and suppressed developmental needs. For her to feel safe enough to do this, she must trust that the therapist is capable of understanding her most profound emotional states (Clark, 1991). As the relationship deepens, the therapist will use more advanced empathic transactions (Rogers, 1961/1967), and since there is no such thing as "the

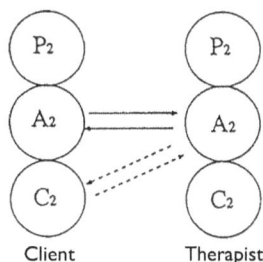

Figure 4.4 The Empathic Transaction.

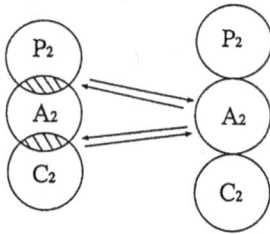

Figure 4.5 Responding to the Patient's Felt Meaning.

immaculate perception," empathy will involve the therapist's imaginative use of self.

Kohut (1984) defined empathy as "the capacity to think and feel oneself into the life of another person" (p. 82). Rycroft (1995) defines empathy as "the capacity to put oneself into the other's shoes" (p. 47). Empathy is, therefore, a combination of skill and technique and a reflection of who we are and how we are ourselves. Before we can imaginatively immerse ourselves in another's experiences, we need to have an empathic relationship with our own Child ego state since it will be our use of our own process that will most inform how we understand someone else.

For example, if I have an empathic relationship with my own despairing Child, I will be more likely to recognize and tolerate this state in my patient and not try to resolve or change it into something else. Thus, empathy involves the therapist in an introspective process in which she is required to use herself imaginatively, allowing time for reflection and being prepared to share her understanding of the patient as a type of offering for consideration rather than as a fact or a theoretical certainty.

Empathic Inquiry: One variant of the empathic transaction is the process of attuned inquiry described by Erskine (1993). He argues that the therapist needs to begin by assuming that he or she does not know about the patient and therefore respectfully seeks to understand the patient's subjective experience. Not only will the therapist listening empathically, as already described, but he or she will be open to exploration from a place of genuine inquiry. The patient and therapist will thus co-construct the meaning of the patient's subjective experience as it emerges from the combination of empathic understanding and inquiry. This communication also allows trust to develop as the patient experiences the therapist's respect for and genuine interest in her innermost psychological experiences.

Empathic transactions and empathic inquiry need to continue throughout the deconfusion phase to provide an "Aumbrella" of empathic ambience to the transferential relationship. We emphasize the use of empathy when making any intervention and suggest that empathy provides the container for the therapeutic relationship. We do not mean that empathy means we should always "get it right" for the patient or that we never confront. With the best will in the world, it is still not possible to understand completely someone else. Paradoxically, it may be that in feeling misunderstood, the patient moves to a deeper understanding of herself. For instance, understanding our patient's frustrations with us for our limitations, or hearing our patient's anger with us when we unwittingly rupture the empathic relationship, or trying to understand a patient's apparently incomprehensible annoyance with us is, in our view, a part of empathic understanding.

Step Two: The Transferential Relationship

There are many definitions of transference, which, when loosely summarized, suggest that it describes the patient's emotional attitude toward the psychotherapist. In deconfusion, the patient attempts to communicate within the context of the therapeutic relationship unarticulated experience of which she is unaware of, that is, reproduce unmet needs and early relationship patterns and experiences in the relationship with the therapist. It is a type of "inarticulate speech of the heart" (Morrison, 1983) that communicates to the therapist through behavior and coded language what cannot be verbalized directly. Many clinicians will recognize the increasing number of patients who present with this type of disturbance, which can best be understood as a disorder of the self that shows itself most commonly in narcissistic and borderline traits. In this context, a useful definition of transference is supplied by Stolorow, Brandchaft, and Atwood (1987): "Transference is conceived ... as the expression of a universal psychological striving to organize experience and construct meanings" (p. 46).

We view transference as the vehicle by which the therapist finds out about the unconscious aspects of the patient. "The neurological evidence simply suggests that selective absence of emotion is a problem. Welltargeted and welldeployed emotion seems to be a support system without which the edifice of reason cannot operate properly" (Damasio, 1999, p. 43). These findings seem to suggest that it is untenable to separate feelings from emotions, and further, that feelings are inextricably linked to reasoning. Damasio's research on the brain demonstrates how feeling is always present, although not necessarily conscious. Research by Schore (1994) indicates that the links between feelings and thought is developed in right brain-left brain connections. It therefore seems logical to assume that the emotional availability of the therapist is central to an understanding of the unconscious. Understood in this context, the transferential relationship becomes the gateway to the unconscious. Drawing on the work of Menaker (1995), we have identified three domains of transferential phenomenon. We develop

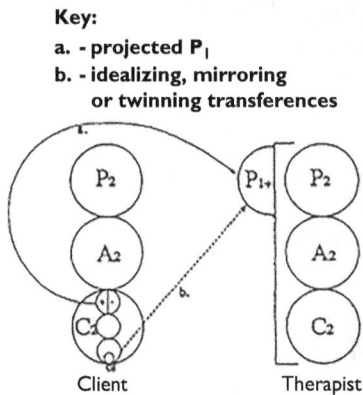

Figure 4.6 Projective and Introjective Transferences (Based on Moiso 1985).

Moiso's (1985) transference model to distinguish between the three types of transference (Figure 4.6) as follows:

1 *Introjective Transference (C$_o$ longings):* In this type of transference, the patient seeks to enter a symbiosis (Schiff et al., 1975) with the therapist to meet developmental needs (C$_o$). "Introjection is both a defense and a normal developmental process; a defense because it diminishes separation anxiety, a developmental process because it renders the subject increasingly autonomous" (Rycroft, 1995, p. 87). Neuroscientists confirm this perspective when they describe how genetic systems program the development of the brain and are activated and influenced by the quality of the infant/environment relationship. When such a relationship is problematic, the person is left with an undeveloped sense of self because important structures in the brain are left unactivated (Schore, 1994). The undeveloped self is, therefore, unable to be autonomous until certain structures in the brain are activated through the relationship. This neuroscientific research provides us with a context in which to understand the psychological need for a transferential relationship.

Kohut (1971) described the emergence of archaic needs for symbiosis in the therapeutic relationship as self-object transferences. He understood the development of such transferences as attempts by the patient to get his self-object needs met. The term "self-object" refers to a group of psychological functions that enables a person to maintain self experience. When these needs are thwarted in the infant he will continue as a grown up to try and get these needs met in the environment. They include the following:

Mirror Transference: The mirror transference involves two types of transferring. One is the mergermirroring transference, a complete firstorder symbiosis (Schiff et al., 1975) in which the therapist is experienced as a part of the patient's grandiose self (Co and Po). For such patients, who experience the need for prolonged self-involvement, the therapist's subjectivity can feel, at best, irrelevant, and, at worst, an intrusive rupturing of the therapeutic need to be fully and completely heard without interruption.

The other type of mirror transference occurs when the therapist is perceived as separate and the patient seeks her approval and admiration. The patient has a need to be mirrored for something she recognizes as authentic so she feels seen, met, and understood.

Idealizing Transference: If there has been too early a rupture in the child's perception of his powerful adult, this unconscious need to participate in the strength and calm of the "perfect" other will communicate itself in the idealized transference. Such ruptures occur either because circumstances are unfavorable, such as the mother's postpartum depression or a bereavement in the family, or for reasons of parental ineptitude, which can range from misattunement to physical and emotional abuse. A significant amount of therapy involves dealing with some trauma and associated aspects of disassociation. A central feature of posttraumatic stress is that there is a realization that no adult is powerful enough to stop dreadful things from happening: Illusions are shattered. After trauma there is a need to reconstruct illusion: "I'm important, you are omnipotent: The world is a safe place." The idealizing transference enables the patient to occupy a state of illusion, a creation of the Garden of Eden before the Fall. From this position, which in such cases was prematurely interrupted, the patient can be assisted to assimilate a more functional reality. The therapist, of course, must be able to let go of the idealization when the patient is ready. Otherwise the patient is infantilized indefinitely and never learns to deal with the empowering experience of handling betrayal and disillusionment, which ultimately can lead to maturity and the possibility for growth.

Twinship: The twinship transference refers to what might be called fellow feelings, a sense that we are like others. The child wants to "do what mummy does." She wants to identify and take part in the big world. In this transferential domain, the therapist will feel a pull from her patient to affirm a sense of essential sameness. The self-object need is for the patient to feel validated and to experience a sense of belonging and connectedness so that she can develop her mix of intelligence and talents into usable skills.

2   *Projective Transferences (P_{1+}/P_{1-})—The Defensive Transferences:* The selfobject transferences do not quite explain the projections of the patient onto the therapist. We think that these features, when displayed in the transference, are better understood in terms of projective or defensive transference. It is, of course, possible for both transferences to

overlap. While still wanting merger experiences, the patient may also need the therapist to contain and deal with projections. In this transferential domain, the patient projects P_{1+}/P_{1-} onto the therapist in order to work through unintegrated experiences. "Owing to the influence of Melanie Klein, projection has been accepted as a normal developmental process" (Rycroft, 1995, p. 140).

In a misattuned environment, the infant splits between "good" and "bad."

> Splitting of both ego and object tends to be linked with denial and projection, the trio constituting a schizoid defence by which parts of the self (and internal objects) are disowned and attributed to objects in the environment. (p. 173)

The projective transference is the patient's mechanism for keeping a coherent sense of self while projecting repressed internal conflict onto the therapist. Patients who require this transferential experience often flip back and forth between good and bad. The idealizing aspect of this transference is dissimilar from the idealizing merger transference described earlier in that it usually communicates a significant amount of anxiety to the therapist. She knows only too well that the "love" will turn to "hate."

Faced with a patient's anger, it can be helpful to distinguish between at least two different types of negative transference. A patient may feel angry and enraged because the therapist has unwittingly "missed" him or her, and indeed the therapist may well be at fault. Such ruptures, often seen as mistakes, can be very beneficial to the therapy since the patient has an opportunity to connect with deep affective experience and express it, for the first time, in the company of a concerned, caring, and appropriately apologetic other. However, sometimes the negative transference may need to be sustained over a longer period of time to support psychological integration. Winnicott (1949) warned us not to deny our feelings of hate in the countertransference but to find ways to contain them and keep them for interpretation purposes.

If a patient's primary attachment was experienced through hatred, he may have difficulties in attaching securely enough to the therapist to do the work unless he can feel some of that negative charge. This can be a difficult situation for therapists who find it hard to do anything other than feel warm, positive, and sympathetic toward their patients. However, it could be therapeutically ineffective to deny feelings of anger when hatred is attempting to manifest itself in the therapeutic relationship.

3   *Transformational Transferences (C₁) (Projective Identification)* (Figure 4.7): We refer here to the process of projective identification, particularly as it is defined by Ogden (1992), who amplified Klein's (1986) original concept.

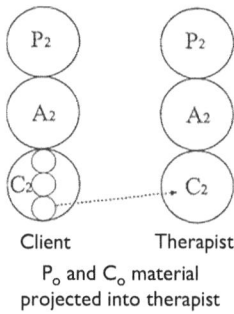

P₂ and C₀ material
projected into therapist

Client   Therapist

Figure 4.7 Transformational Transferences.

Ogden proposed that the infant induces a feeling state in the other that corresponds to a state that he is unable to experience for himself. The recipient allows the induced state to reside within, and by reinternalizing this externally metabolized experience, the infant gains a change in the quality of his experience (Ogden, 1992). In this transference, the therapist is required to transform the experience by making it containable and meaningful. This suggests that the patient's core or splitoff self is "felt" by the therapist, who finds himself containing and feeling something which is hard to identify as "other" than the patient.

Projective Identification is a concept that addresses the way in which feelingstates corresponding to the unconscious fantasies of one person (the projector) are engendered in and processed by another person (the recipient), that is, the way in which one person makes use of another person to experience and contain an aspect of himself.

(Ogden, 1992, p.1)

This suggests to us that the therapist must be receptive to feeling something that she experiences as foreign and yet that clamors for her attention.

Step Three: Examination of Countertransference

Case example: A male patient arrived for group and sat in the therapist's chair. The therapist responded by sitting in another seat while containing feelings of apprehension and some anger. The patient looked slightly uncomfortable but began to boast about his newly acquired "power" and how he was now in the "driver's seat." His manner seemed to show contempt toward the therapist, who began to feel powerless, infuriated, and engulfed by rage. As the session evolved, group members challenged the patient's belief that he was gaining power by sitting in the therapist's seat, and the patient began to look defeated. As her own angry feelings sub-sided, the therapist became aware of feeling powerless and humiliated. Alive to her own distress, the therapist began to imagine how the patient might have felt as a child in some of the situations that he had described from his past. (There was ample historical evidence for a scenario in which the defiant child had provoked an authority figure and been severely beaten and humiliated as a result.) Becoming aware, too, of the potential for humiliation within the group situation, the therapist intervened to make contact with the hurt, distressed, isolated child hidden underneath the grandiose defense. The client's defense evaporated, and he spoke movingly from an authentic place of a painful sense of worthlessness and a profound need for emotional connection. The scene was now set for fur-ther work in deconfusion of the Child.

If we think of the transferential relationship as the interactional field between two people, then the therapist's response within this energy field—commonly known as countertransference—will be significant. Her recep-tivity to her subjective responses to the patient and her willingness to engage with her experience is a central feature in relational psychotherapy. Such a process necessarily involves a type of introspective musing because infor-mation cannot be forced from the unconscious; it only emerges if we allow the space for it.

It is through the transferential process that we as therapists are invited into the unconscious world of our patients. Therefore, a careful examination of our countertransference is vital to the growth and change of mental states within the patient. In the context of a therapeutic relationship, the thera-pist's own primary anxieties will often be provoked. Although this process can feel unsettling and disturbing, it is actually a sign of health in the therapeutic relationship. It may even be the first time that the patient's Child has been able to impact another and have that person remain constant and consistent within the relationship.

It is in this way that our patients seek to use us in order to integrate the unconscious contents of the Child ego state. In therapy, this process follows the same rules and functions as those followed in normal child development. When the mother/other/therapist is good enough, he or she is able to deal with the infant's/patient's frustrated feelings or experiences and help the infant/patient to manage them. This is achieved through a process referred to as "projective identification" (Klein, 1986) but that is also understood by self psychologists (Kohut, 1971) in terms of empathic immersion in oneself in order to understand and help another make sense of his or her experience.

Moiso and Novellino (2000) have argued that in transactional analysis, the "enormous methodological and clinical consequences of accepting and working with the transferential and countertransferential dimensions of transactions" (p. 184) have sometimes been neutralized by considering transference as only one dimension of the therapeutic relationship. They point to Berne's original criticism of psychoanalysis as a theory that was too detached from problems of a phenomenological nature. Transactional analysts gained the phenomenology but were often diverted away from the transferential relationship.

We now seek to redress this balance and argue that by making the transferential relationship central to the work, we have access to an exciting and complex emotional dynamic. In accepting the validity of the therapist's emotional life, we have a rich source of data available to us about the nature of the patient's problems. The three transferential domains outlined earlier can be useful in tracking the therapist's countertransference and supporting treatment direction. For reasons of space we do not explore this further except to indicate some of what the therapist may experience in these transferential domains.

1   *Introjective Transference:* When the therapist is required to be intro-jected or "coopted," then she can be prey at times to feelings of boredom and even sleepiness. The therapist may find that her own narcissistic needs may get in the way, and unless alert to this counter-transferential response, she may insist on her presence in a way that will not be effective in the therapy. If she persists in making interventions, then a Child-Child competition can emerge that is nontherapeutic. At the same time, the therapist will be required to be emotionally attuned so that she is alert to naming and reflecting emotional responses without being intrusive.

2   *Projective Transferences (P_{1+}/P_{1-})—The Defensive Transferences:* These transferences are more reflective of borderline features and disorders. In extreme cases, the therapist will feel as though she is on a roller coaster—up one minute and down the next. In less extreme cases, when she is "up," she will nervously anticipate that the "down" will follow, if not sooner, then later. There is no resting place! The therapist often feels connected with an intense sense of her own vulnerability, since her own primary processes will be stirred up by the volatile interpersonal dynamics. The therapist will often feel under extreme provocation to act out her countertransference, and although apparently calm, she may be tempted to make a particularly "hostile" interpretation under the guise of being "therapeutic."

3   *Transformational Transferences (C_1):* Countertransferential reactions in this domain are diverse and often profound. When the patient projects archaic and unprocessed distress out into the therapeutic environment, the therapist's primary processes will be mobilized. The previous case study conveys some of this experience.

Step Four: Responding to the Patient Using Empathic Interventions

In *Principles of Group Treatment*, Berne (1966/1994, pp. 233258) outlined his "therapeutic operations"—which constitute eight forms of therapist intervention—along with specific instructions about how to use them. The eight operations are: interrogation, specification, confrontation, explanation, illustration, confirmation, and, for deconfusion of the Child ego state, interpretation and crystallization. However, we view this as an artificial split between deconfusion and decontamination. We think that the process of deconfusion is an integral aspect of the therapeutic alliance and therefore begins immediately.

A close reading of these instructions suggests that Berne attended carefully to the transferential relationship without referring to it as such. This demonstrates that he was aware of the skill, sensitivity, and intuition required when choosing how to respond to a patient. For instance, he warned of how an illwishing Parent ego state might misuse an intervention. He also stressed the importance of not humiliating the Child, which again implies his understanding of how easy it can be to misuse these operations if one does not consider the transferential meaning. As highlighted in the last case cited, it can be relatively easy to fall into this trap and offer, for example, an interpretation or confrontation out of unconscious hostility toward the patient. When Berne directed us toward ensuring a valid working alliance with the Adult and the Child, he was implicitly acknowledging the existence of multiple levels within the therapeutic relationship.

We believe that Berne undersold his own excellent theory by presenting it in a somewhat facile way with the result that readers may easily miss the clinical acuity and also the therapeutic care that he manifested. To address this problem, we have articulated our own description of his operations, which we have renamed "empathic interventions."

Since Berne's day, research has indicated time and again that empathy is central to therapeutic understanding (Kohut, 1971; Rogers, 1961/1967), and, indeed, for some, it is the single component in therapy that correlates with a positive outcome (Kirschenbaum & Henderson, 1990). Therefore, we emphasize the use of empathy when making any intervention and suggest that empathy provides the container for the therapeutic relationship. As such, we view empathy as both a cognitive and a feeling process.

We do not mean to imply, however, that empathy requires that we always "get it right" for the patient or that we never confront; rather, we suggest that regardless of the intervention, we make it with a view to understanding how we can best enable the patient to feel understood. Even with the most positive intentions, clearly it is not possible to understand someone else completely. This, in our view, offers empathic understanding in itself. While an effective analysis of the therapist's countertransference provides her with a vast range of information about her patient, we may well ask how we are supposed to use this information.

We have already established that the transferential relationship is at the heart of the therapeutic work. Any methodology will, therefore, arise from an understanding that the therapeutic work must be firmly embedded in the relationship between therapist and patient. For us, the meaning of such a relationship resides in the fact that there are two subjectivities brought together in the relationship. Not only the person who is the therapist matters but also his or her personal history, capacity for emotional involvement, empathic understanding, and skill for relatedness will shape the therapy. Thus, we believe that it is the sensibility of the therapist that matters; not a set of techniques. The defining feature of this work resides in the therapist's capacity for continuing sensitivity, and it is this that will inform the prowess and incisiveness or otherwise of her interventions.

In proposing the following set of techniques, therefore, we are aware that they will, of necessity, need to be adopted and adapted by the therapist to become part of his style and way of working. In other words, we are suggesting that a technique is not powerful in and of itself, nor does it carry any extra weight except in the sense of how and when the therapist chooses to use it. Instead, we propose the use of empathic interventions as a way of accessing these deeper states of experience. The techniques are: inquiry, specification, confrontation, explanation, illustration, confirmation, interpretation, crystallization, holding, invitation, selfdisclosure, and echoing (R. Little, personal communication, June 2000). Because of the dictates of space, we limit our description of these empathic interventions as follows:

Inquiry and specification: The first two operations described by Berne are interrogation and specification, which we referred to in the section entitled "Step One: The Empathic Transaction." We prefer the word "inquiry" to "interrogation," in part because of the unfortunate link between the word "interrogation" and forms of stressful examination. Inquiry is a gentler word, one usually associated with phenomenological inquiry, and it encompasses the sensitive exploration of all ego states (Erskine, 1991; Erskine & Trautmann, 1996). This intervention is also very much an expression of the therapist's identity. He will ask those questions of the patient that make the most sense to him. Specification, we believe, is a type of accurate empathy that can include the more advanced empathy outlined in step one. The therapist's way of organizing and understanding his emotional experience will fundamentally influence what and how he chooses to use this intervention.

Explanation and interpretation: Throughout this chapter, we have stressed the importance of empathic understanding of the patient's feelings and attitudes. However, this alone is insufficient. It is important to assist the patient ultimately in making sense of her experience in therapy. While it may be healing to feel and express an unmet need or emotion, without understanding and integration, a patient may be doomed to play and replay her reenactment of the past. An important part of this process of integration is explanation and interpretation. Knowing when to offer these interventions is not easy. Meaning needs to emerge through the relationship; it is articulated through a process of empathic resonance and will require decoding.

Explanation attempts to describe in Adult terms the dynamics of the patient's experience. It can relate to any situations and relationships in the patient's life and refers to previously specified material. An example might be: "So, when other car drivers hoot at you, for a moment you are aware of a scared Child ego state, and then you kick straight into Parent and think, 'They're going to pay for that!'"

Interpretation involves trying to find a voice for the Child. It is an attempt to "decode and detoxify" (Berne, 1966/1994, p. 243) the patient's communications. An example might be, "You say you think I will reject you. I think that when you showed your mother how much you needed her, she pushed you away. It must be frightening to let yourself make me important." Thus, interpretation is not simply organizing what is known between therapist and patient; it is giving a voice to a part of the patient that seems to her to be literally unspeakable. This deepens the Adult's understanding of her own self.

We are intrigued with Berne's use of the word "detoxify," which we believe encapsulates an important factor in the process of deconfusing the Child. At a fundamental level the Child can feel shamed and terrified by the strength of her need for mirroring or for an idealized other and by the feelings that she decided were unacceptable when she was developing her script. She can feel "toxic" and may consequently fight against allowing her mirroring or idealizing transferences to emerge clearly in the relationship with their concomitant neediness or natural rage if they are thwarted. She may use all manner of other strategies to have contact and feel OK without revealing the depths of her yearnings.

Transactional analysis offers us excellent ways of understanding these defensive strategies (e.g., games [Berne, 1964]; racketeering [English, 1976]; and passive behavior [Schiff et al., 1975]). If the therapist were to meet these defensive strategies with affective empathy alone, the patient might feel good, but she would not necessarily change her script. For therapy to be successful there must be an increase in understanding and selfcontainment. This involves explanation and interpretation on the part of the therapist.

Nevertheless, we reiterate our original point. We have found that interpretation is therapeutically more effective when empathic resonance is maintained. Comprehension without compassion for self does nothing to detoxify the patient's position in relation to her Child. We believe that understanding, which can include naming and voicing the meaning of the dynamics, is one of the deepest forms of empathy.

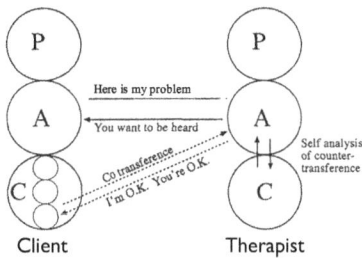

Figure 4.8 The Therapeutic Transaction.

Figure 4.8 shows the therapeutic transaction. The arrows from the therapist's Adult into her own C_1 indicate her use of her own Child ego states to analyze her countertransference and to help her choose one of the empathic interventions.

Three Additional Operations

Holding: Knowing when it is appropriate to offer an explanation or an interpretation is a constant challenge. It is important to be aware that sometimes the patient simply needs "holding" instead of explanation or interpretation or indeed any intervention aimed at doing more than offering the steady containing presence of a nonjudgmental therapist who is perceived as having the potency to offer the protection and permission needed. We refer here to a metaphorical holding within the energy field of the relationship rather than a physical holding. Slochower (1966) described three major times when this type of holding is essential: (1) when the patient has regressed to total dependence; (2) when the patient's need for mirroring is absolute and anything other than affirmation and empathy would seem like an attack; and (3) when the patient is connected with P_{1-} rage and hate and any attempt to explain or interpret could be experienced as punishing, rejecting, or irrelevant.

Invitation: It can be appropriate to encourage the patient to voice her feelings and thoughts about the therapist. This encouragement can take the form of an explicit invitation or by the therapist noticing and commenting on the patient's nonverbal reactions to the therapist's interventions. A particular form of invitation can be used when the patient reconnects with repressed feelings stored in P_{1-}. Such feelings can threaten a cohesive sense of self and are therefore projected onto the therapist to relieve the patient and restore equilibrium in the Child.

At these points, it can be useful to accept the projection as if it were true and invite the patient to explain how the therapy could be improved (Epstein & Feiner, 1979). This offers the patient the opportunity to reintegrate the repressed experience at a nonthreatening pace. For example, if the therapist can survive an angry attack without becoming hostile or accept the account of his imperfections with equanimity, he models a way of containing what is most threatening and engulfing for the patient.

Self-disclosure of the countertransference: Sometimes the therapist may decide to offer an account of her countertransference to her patient, even when the feelings may be difficult or uncomfortable. This can be a form of empathic understanding of the original protocol. The therapist is, in a sense, offering back the projected material, which makes the timing of the intervention crucial. Berne did not often suggest that a psychotherapist share his own responses. However, we believe that the decision to talk about one's countertransference in order to illuminate the dynamics and link them to the patient's childhood can sometimes be the most empathic response possible. It can also open up the possibility of examining the cocreation of the experience in the therapeutic relationship. This means the therapist is willing to reveal her own attitudes in order to explore how she might be contributing to the patient's experience.

While we have expanded the operations by adding three interventions to the list, we have omitted confrontation, illustration, confirmation, and crystallization here. We believe that they, too, can be extremely valuable in the deconfusion process and will explore them more in future publications.

Conclusion

We have offered a model of psychotherapy using an analytic approach grounded in transactional analysis. In doing so, we have been influenced by transactional analysts such as Haykin (1980), Moiso (1985), Novellino (1984), Clark (1991), Blackstone (1993), Erskine (1991, 1993, 1994), and Shmukler (1991). We have developed our model from the structural model of ego states to provide a theoretical basis that includes a theory of the self. We have emphasized the importance of the transferential relationship as the vehicle through which deconfusion of the Child is achieved. In addition, we have offered an imaginative development of Berne's therapeutic operations as the basis for the methodology. We believe that this work offers significant theoretical implications for transactional analysts wishing to work with indepth consideration of the Child ego state.

REFLECTIONS

This chapter forms the basis of the move away from classical TA towards a transactional analysis of the unconscious processes and forms the core base of what was to become the book *Transactional Analysis: A Relational Perspective* (Hargaden & Sills, 2002). The theoretical concept of domains of transference was recognized by the International Transactional Analysis Association when we won the 2007 Eric Berne Memorial Award. We began our research with this chapter followed by the book after a series of conversations about the difficulty many trainees and supervises seemed to have with "fitting" their work into the theoretical perspectives of Classical, Redecision, and Cathexis transactional analysis. Our conversations hinged on the fact that many clinicians were clearly doing effective work with their clients and yet there was no theoretical perspective, which enabled them to synthesize their experience with a theoretical perspective. As cited in the chapter, we found some literature in transactional analysis, such as the valuable contributions made by Moiso and Novellino (2000), which enabled us to introduce a different paradigm. Their work along with some others helped us to move away from trying to "make sense of things' towards looking into the deeper meanings contained within a multiplicity of transferential processes. This brought the focus for clinicians onto the unconscious states, both within the client and also themselves. There was therefore an implicit requirement that clinicians find a therapeutic relationship where they could do this work for themselves.

This transferential paradigm opened up the possibility for the clinician to value her feelings, intuition, sensations, and her imaginative responses to the narratives she was listening to. Although we did not know it at the time, we were giving the green light to our institutions, trainees and supervises to begin a process of valuing non linear knowledge. Schore, Damasio, McGilchrist, and others have focussed our minds on the significance of the right hemisphere of the brain. When having these conversations at the time of developing our theoretical framework both Charlotte (Sills) and I had been in Jungian analysis, which had enabled us to value our intuitive, feeling and sensitive minds that we had both inherited but had learned to automatically disown as irrelevant. Learning about ourselves in this deeper more connected way, valuing our very intuitive, feeling minds, we then turned our attention into what we now understand as a synthesizing process of linking this knowledge to the left hemisphere. We began to organize therapeutic experience by using information from multiple theoretical sources. It was collating and distributing this knowledge that we were now valuing that took us on a theoretical journey towards the domains of transference.

Throughout the book *Transactional Analysis: A Relational Perspective*, there are many references to songs and poetry. For instance, "I want you to hurt like I do" by Randy Newman is the subtitle we use for countertransference. These lyrics help us to decode the client's professed meaning and to recognize how the transference really needs to be received by the therapist. Likewise, "Tangled Up in Blue" by Bob Dylan captures the paradoxical nature of how the therapist gets caught up in the countertransference. "The Inarticulate Speech of the Heart" by Van Morrison evokes the very nature of what it is we are trying to do as psychotherapists as we listen, hear, decode and translate to the best of our abilities. We end with Dylan's "Things have changed" which is in part a rather ironic gesture to those theory makers who don't want to change but stick religiously to the received wisdom of what it as they originally learned. However, if theory is to mean anything, it has to be alive, breathing, and open to evolving. In the 20 years since writing, this I have changed to rethinking transference as a type of bidirectionality of the relational unconscious that-transference may be understood as intersubjectivity. These are all different descriptions that can fit the emotional and psychological process that occurs between therapist and client. Whatever we call these processes, however, has to be linked to theoretical understanding. In order to evolve, we need to continue to link in with multiple perspectives and not stick rigidly with one way of looking at our minds.

Chapter 5

"Come On You Blues! Fathers"

Paper presented at Relational TA Conference hosted by the Metanoia Institute, February 2006

Helena Hargaden

For reasons of confidentiality I will keep information about the group and the two individuals I focus on to a minimum. I have changed their details so that they will not be recognised and have permission to use the information I share.

"What is on your minds and hearts this warm summer evening?" I asked. I had barely finished when Pierre announced excitedly that he had something to share with the group and that he needed their help. He told us that he had had an unexpected telephone call from his father in Paris requesting that Pierre fly over that weekend to help his father sort out a technical problem with a new digital television. He was unsure how to respond, he was nervous, he was excited, he was worried—he did not know what to do. "Of course you should go," I thought. "The man is crying out to talk with you because you rowed last time, but he couches it in some techno babble because he cannot say what he really thinks and feels." Although I knew more details about Pierre's dynamic with his father than the group members, because he also saw me individually, I was rather astounded by the group's response. Stuff his father, seemed to be the general consensus. He was arrogant and out of order to expect Pierre to down tools and take a plane to Paris just to fix a stupid TV. Eventually, a group member, who had been silent up until then, wondered if his father might be offering an olive branch. I relaxed. I observed that Pierre responded only to this comment. It became clear that there was no question that he would not go, but he wished the group to help him because he was liable to lose his temper with his irascible father, whose failing health made it difficult for him to tolerate any frustrations. I could see that some members of the group had not understood what was happening and so I decided to translate his father's request into the language of emotional literacy. I said that his father really meant, my lovely son, I am so sorry about the last time we met, I want to be with you and spend time with you before I die, and to let you know I love you. And I value what you give me. Pierre warmed to this; by voicing it I brought his feeling into the realm of a thought. One group member, however, still looked rather septical.

DOI: 10.4324/9781032266237-6

Matteus had been separated from his mother immediately after birth for about nine months, because his mother had been seriously ill. I sometimes fancied I could feel the "fierce stare of the infant" so poignantly described by Erikson on a visit to a nursery of abandoned babies. Matteus' later relationship with his mother was intense but highly unsatisfactory. She seemed to have a rather macho style of parenting, humiliating, taunting, and "hardening" him up as a boy; and, at times, was somewhat sexually inappropriate with him. Not surprisingly, Matteus had a deeply distrustful feeling towards women; yet, struggled with his desire and need for them. We had had a bumpy relationship which had often threatened to prematurely abrupt, but one that had become increasingly rewarding for us both. Although I was aware of the "fierce stare" feeling I often had with Matteus, I paid it no attention. Instead, I was preoccupied with Pierre who had managed to capture my sole attention.

Pierre now laughingly responded to my "translation" saying it was well known that men were from Mars and women from Venus. Getting really into the mood I remarked how some men seemed to use a ball, as in football, as a way of expressing a wide variety of feelings. When Pierre laughed and agreed, I felt further encouraged to develop my theme; and when it turned out that the digital TV was required in order for his father to access the sports channel so he could watch some protracted football tournament (quite possibly the World Cup), I segued into comic exaggeration. The warm evening, thoughts of my holiday, and the friendly and warm exchange I was having had seemingly gone to my head. It was almost as though I was having a laugh with a friend in a café or bar. But not entirely.

This incident created a vibrant stir throughout the group, which led to lively and deep exchanges. Given the group setting, there were multiple meanings relating to this enactment for both Pierre and the group. However, I will focus on my relationship with Matteus. He was furious with me, telling me that I was not taking into consideration the fact that men had been hunters, were biologically primed for different tasks, and, therefore, expressed their feelings differently. I was quite shocked by the extent of his anger, and for an instant felt overwhelmed and unable to think. I felt cornered and misunderstood. I felt angry with him that he was making this into a gender war when that had not been my intention. A part of me felt stimulated into arguments about gender inequality; but in another part of me, I could hear desperate searing pain behind these words and I knew we could not work it through in the group. Although I was able to be involved in deeply affective interpersonal contact with the rest of the group, with Matteus, this was impossible—feelings were running too deep. I looked forward instead to seeing him later in the week.

At our next individual session he came in and smiled at me. I felt relieved and smiled back, but it turned out to be short lived. He told me that he was furious with me because he felt that I was not owning up to my contempt for men; that he had felt humiliated and not heard by me at all when he had pointed to the existence of biological differences between men and women. He thought that my expectation that men express their feelings in the same way as women was sexist and that he felt betrayed by me. I felt most uncomfortable and completely misunderstood for the meaning he was attributing to my feelings was not resonating for me. I did not hate men. My father had been a lyrical type of man, not macho, and, although inadequate in his parenting, not someone whom I had hated. Indeed, I had recovered my deep love for him during my own therapeutic journey. Nor did I disagree with Matteus about men and women expressing their feelings differently and having different relational patterns. As a lifelong feminist, I had fought for the rights of women; but, in the past 15 years, had become increasingly sensitive to how boys and men suffered as a result of gender inequality. This was partly as a consequence of having two sons but I had also become interested in how men's relational patterns were subtly pathologised by psychotherapy.

However, I thought it would be therapeutically ineffective to argue or placate Matteus out of his experience by getting into the facts of the argument or to say he had misunderstood my intention, so I tried to stay with him. I referred him back to his mother's hostile and humiliating parenting, her inappropriate sexual responses, which had made him feel so powerless, and his underlying rage with all women. But Matteus would have none of it.

"It's not my mother—it is you!" he said.

I struggled between wanting to fight with him, and trying to think about the meaning of what was happening. I said, I found it hard to understand exactly why he felt so enraged with me, given that we had discussed it in the group and referred to some interpretations that had emerged, which had been insightful and deepening for others in the group. Did none of that mean anything to him? I wondered if he had found my attitude towards football offensive but he laughed derisively and said that he couldn't care less about football that he was a cricket man. This threw me completely because for me it was something about football. I looked at the clock; we were half way through the session and completely steeped in impasse. Nothing I said had made any difference. He was not listening to me. I found him aggressive and I thought he was being unreasonable. But I had to find a way of reaching him. He was reaching out to me. After all, he had come to the session to tell me about his feelings; and still, somehow, *I was not getting it.*

In his paper on enactment, amusingly and pertinently entitled, "Dumb Spots, Blind Spots and Hard Spots," McLaughlin (2005) refers reassuringly to the ubiquity of enactment within the therapeutic dialogue. "Enactment in a broad sense can be construed in all the behaviours of both parties in the analytic relationship" (McLaughlin, 2005, p. 186). It makes sense, in the rarefied and intense atmosphere of the therapeutic relationship, that there will be an "enormous intensification of the appeal or manipulative intent of our words and silences" (McLaughlin, 2005, p. 187). From McLaughlin's perspective, the word, enactment, within the analytic situation, suggests a purposeful interplay of at least two parties. Thus, enactment involves an interactive process, which McLaughlin (p. 189) describes, more specifically, as "referring to events occurring within the dyad that both parties experience as being the consequence of behaviour in the other." McLaughlin's perspective is firmly embedded in a two-person psychology:

> These charged words of the analytic dialogue are themselves embedded in and surcharged by a steady clamour of nonverbal communication between the pair, much of what is registered and processed, at times subliminally, by both parties. (p. 187)

From such a perspective, the subjectivity of the therapist becomes more of a focal point than if we are merely to describe the therapist as having a countertransference. In other words, what about the subjectivity and auto-biographical elements the therapist brings to the therapeutic encounter?

In the classical tradition of transactional analysis, enactments are under-stood as a game. A game involves a series of transactions, which are initially complementary, until a switch occurs, when participants experience momen-tary confusion. It used to be thought that the therapist must guard against a game, asking themselves, not if I am in a game, but what game am I in? and then bring it to closure, reverting to Adult to Adult transactions. However, in 1983, Moiso introduced the idea of game enactments as therapeutically useful; that if we interrupt it too early, we prevent gaining further information about the patient's unconscious process. In our book on relational TA, Charlotte Sills and I take this further, describing transference as not a path-ological process alone, but a normal one; and delineate three domains of transferential phenomenon to describe the plurality and complexity of relatedness. We portray the therapeutic relationship as the backdrop for a complex web of other relationships, which are happening, often at an implicit level of consciousness:

> It is the responsibility of the psychotherapist to acknowledge, recognize, and hear the drumbeat of her own inarticulate heart longings, in the service of understanding the communication from her patient.
> (Hargaden & Sills, 2002, pp. 47–48)

You will remember that I left our therapeutic couple in a rather uncomfortable position—both sitting, feeling angry with each other, misunderstood, and hurt. We were half way through the session and nothing that I had said had made any difference. I had to take my own advice and hear the drumbeat of my own inarticulate heart longings in an attempt to understand Matteus.

As I had this thought I began to associate and had an image of a two-year-old boy with callipers on his leg. It was my father. He had had polio as a child and, sitting there now, it suddenly made sense to me that of course, he had been unable to play football as a child. He may well have felt an outsider in his own home town of Bray, in county Wicklow, even before he left for London and experienced the isolating life of an immigrant. Meeting my mother, they both lived in Ireland for six years before deciding to live in Liverpool with their young family, where he was further cast as an outsider by his accent; his attitude; and, still, the effects of the polio, manifest in his limp, always making him look a little drunk in his gait—so fitting neatly with the stereotype of the drunken Irishman that he fought against all his life. I was back in the schoolyard, surrounded by kids, "Who do you support – Everton or Liverpool?" I was new—an immigrant, I was frightened and felt bullied by them. There was a religious association to each team, one was Catholic and the other Protestant, and I was never sure which team was which; but the answer mattered because serious allegiance to not only football but God were at stake. He must have had similar experiences. My father dealt with his pain and confusion by referring to them all as bigots, idiots, and other choice phrases that I cannot repeat here. He communicated his painful sense of exclusion to me by mocking those to whom he could not belong, an experience which I absorbed as a part of my self. I could see how his scornful attitude and his attempts to "rise above it" were a defense against the painful feelings aroused by exclusion and not belonging. These thoughts and feelings passed through my mind in about two minutes but, as you all know, that can feel like a long time in the therapeutic situation. Did Matteus sense my struggle? According to Ferenzi (1932), from his lifelong work with traumatised patients, stereotyped compassionate phrases expressed by the psychotherapist fail to connect emotionally with the patient. He thought that only the genuine emotional experience of the therapist could steer the therapy in a healing direction.

"I think you have a point," I said.

> There *was* something contemptuous in my tone that I was not aware of until you pointed it out. I am not exactly sure what it refers to but it is not exactly what you think it is. For me, I think it is somehow connected with my father, his polio, our exclusion from belonging in Liverpool and the symbolism of that in sport, particularly about football for me.

Tried to choose my words carefully; I knew my thoughts were a bit jumbled but my feelings were evident in my tone. He looked at me quietly in his searching way. At first, nothing. He looked at me closely and then very slowly, he said, "well, that changes everything, I feel warm towards you" and he smiled in a painful sort of way. I was initially alarmed, wondering if my disclosure had made him care too much for me, but he then went on, with tears in his eyes, to make several deep and relevant connections and interpretations about his relationship with his mother, recalling a particularly gruelling incident in which he had been cruelly taunted and humiliated, by the end of which he was sobbing. I had a deep feeling of mutuality with Matteus and could hear the lines of Larkin's poem in my mind: *They fuck you up your mum and dad. They mean not mean to but they do*. I could not remember the rest of the lines but Matteus and I were once again connected.

I would like to take a few minutes now to examine the clinical meaning and effects of my disclosure and the intense emotional interaction between Matteus and I. Firstly, I think that maybe we could say Matteus was ready to discover my subjectivity and that some enactment was necessary for this to happen.

Secondly, I think my attitude towards my disclosure was important in that I was clearly genuinely struggling to find the right words and to contain my own painful feelings. It confirmed his sense of *emotional reality* and allowed for a different meaning to emerge in the here and now relationship. I was a woman, who was not feeling the contempt his mother had once implicitly and explicitly expressed towards him, but was feeling a separate sense of painful feelings. By having an honest and intense emotional interaction with me his emotion was recognised, but not his fantasies. This is very significant as it is well established by those involved in neuroscience (Schore, Siegal, Damasio et al.) that emotion functions as a central organiser and integrator of experience by providing incoming stimuli with specific meaning and motivational direction.

Thirdly, I think this new and different experience of self with other lead him directly into a process of reflection in which he was able to recognise his sense of isolation and feelings of abandonment with a mother who had not only initially abandoned him but who was also misattuned to his sexuality and gender.

Fourthly, it established my openness and honesty because a central and ongoing issue was one of trust. The self disclosure broke through an impasse that had been brewing for a while and took us both into a deeper level of relatedness.

Fifthly, in sharing with him, I showed that I was not so different from him; that I too had sorrow from misguided parenting. That I had both been loved and damaged by my parent, just as he had.

Finally, this disclosure clarified for him the nature of his impact on others; he often gets into a rage with women, perceiving them as manipulative. This key transformative moment brought into his awareness that his rage might be misplaced, and that it could be contained.

Overall, we could say Matteus found his mind through my mind; through my sharing of my mental processes he discovered me and, in doing so, discovered himself. That in this process he developed his capacity for reflective functioning, which, according to Fonagy, is an unconscious process, which lends shape and coherence to self organisation and enables us to distinguish inner from outer reality. Fonagy refers to this process as mentalisation.

Finally, I wish to further comment upon my dumb spots, blind spots, and hard spots. Like McLaughlin, Aron agrees that our own therapy does not mean that we know what is in our unconscious. Although I have been involved in a deep engagement with my therapist for 15 years who has helped me to become more conscious of the transgenerational losses of the Irish diaspora, you can clearly see that this was no guarantee against elements within my unconscious that are beyond my control. But instead of feeling downhearted about this, I feel refreshed to think that we can never fully understand ourselves. I believe this may guard against us becoming jaded and burnt out. How can we ever know ourselves fully?

Some say there is no therapy without the therapist changing in some way. I was certainly changed by this experience; and even as I write, I am aware of a more conscious sense of pain around my father where I feel the echoes of the painful sense of abandonment and exclusion that I both absorbed from him and experienced myself. Recently, I took him from his nursing home in Liverpool to his local pub, which was normally empty in the early afternoon, and where we usually had a quiet drink and listened to Irish songs on the jukebox. On this day, it was full of men and smoke. There was a match showing on the TV. Dad looked pleased. I was surprised. I could not believe it—it was Liverpool playing Everton. The pub was full of men, drinking. I sat down. My father was beside me in his wheelchair. A great growl circulated around the pub, apparently another missed goal! He cannot speak very loudly now but he looked as though he was trying to join in. He gesticulated to the men in an attempt to communicate something but, sadly, both he as an old man in a wheelchair and I as a woman were invisible to them. I bent my head close to him to show him I was listening. "Come on you Blues" he said, and smiled mischievously at me. My father, at last, belonged!

REFLECTIONS

This talk was based on a young man who was with me for only a short time; but he had a significant emotional impact on me as recounted in the talk. I gave this talk at a meeting for IARTA. IARTA was founded on the basis of relational TA and sought to promote relational thinking which went across the board, including psychoanalysis and humanistic psychotherapies. The client in the chapter whom I called Matteus seemed to simmer with hostility but, at the same time, managed to seem invisible on some level. From Eastern Europe, he was an immigrant and it was unclear what was so difficult for him.

As recounted in the article, I "tried" very hard to connect with him and to meet him on any level. As you will see, none of it worked until I had to face my own suffering through the love of my father who was an Irish immigrant. "Sadness and empathy are highly correlated" (McGilchrist, 2009 p. 55). It was only when I made a connection with Matteus that I began to have feeling, which, on some level, I was wanting to avoid, hence my clichéd response to him. When Lear cries, "Is there any cause in nature that makes these hard hearts?" McGilchrist (ibid) says yes, "a defect in the right prefrontal cortex" (p. 86).

As I reflect now on this chapter, I think of of Dylan's epiphanic song "I Pity the Poor Immigrant." The song is a lament for the immigrant's life—the immigrant who is looking for a better life but feels very attached still to his country of origin. It is full of paradox and a type of judgement. The song captures the contradictory nature of the "poor immigrant," which is something I felt as I sat with Matteus. I think it was on some unconscious level that this therapy recalled to me my father's experience. He never felt that he truly belonged and felt, at times, persecuted for being Irish by some people—not everyone! He eventually came to appreciate the land to which he had immigrated, which had offered him a better life in so many ways (see chapter 15 on the Irish Uprising). The title of this talk is a metaphor for joining in, belonging, and becoming part of the community and in this case it meant my father joining in to chant support for the local football team. Maybe Matteus had some sense of this appreciation and an experience of belonging to himself and therefore to the community in our moments of meeting.

Chapter 6

The Anniversary of the Wailing Woman

Helena Hargaden

It was a bright sunny morning in May 2017. I was driving from the south coast of England to the Metanoia Institute in West London. Well, that was the plan but, as you will see, things went a little awry.

It was my first visit since I left the institute in 2009. Metanoia had been my professional base since 1985. My initial training was in person-centred counselling, followed by TA and Gestalt, culminating in my qualification in integrative psychotherapy in 1992. I went on to qualify as a teaching and supervising transactional analyst. From 1989 onwards, I have also been involved in developing the relational turn in transactional analysis, incorporating psychoanalytic and Jungian ideas within a humanistic framework. As a result, relational transactional analysis is now the accepted title and syllabus for the MSc in transactional analysis at the Metanoia Institute. From 1992 to 2009, I taught on various courses at Metanoia and developed the syllabus along relational theoretical lines. In total, I was attached to the organisation for 29 years.

In 2011, I had founded the transgenerational forum with my colleague Maya Wallfisch. Because of this, the director of transactional analysis at the Metanoia Institute had invited me to teach on the "Options" weekend, the theme of which was trauma. Options referred to the weekend in which trainees could choose which course they wanted.

The Metanoia Institute

The Metanoia Institute was founded by Petruska Clarkson, Sue Fish, and Brian Dobson. Well educated in integrative systems of psychology and psychiatry, they began their educational project in very modest circumstances, starting with therapy and training groups in one of the rooms in their shared apartment. Their groups became very popular in a short space of time and, before long, the organisation moved into an impressive set of houses in South West London. They were expansive in their teaching methods, experimental, knowledgeable, and philosophically broad in their applications.

DOI: 10.4324/9781032266237-7

Not only were they highly qualified, they brought with them alternative cultural views. Coming from South Africa, and as informed and liberal people, they were, of course, anti-apartheid. At the same time, they offered cultural ways of thinking that seemed exciting because for many of us, they were new and even daring. For instance, I think my first set of notes that I made when I began my training, was to: (a) get a cleaner, (b) have regular massage, (c) make sure I took adequate holidays, and so the list went on. The sense of entitlement from their privileged backgrounds was unashamedly passed on to us and this was refreshing. No hair shirts for their trainees in psychotherapy! They understood that in order to give in a healthy way, you needed optimum self care and that this needed to be top of our list alongside regular psychotherapy and supervision. These suggestions were made long before any type of regulation was in place. To this day, I recall these "instructions" for health, and they have enabled me to have a long and successful career by translating the concrete instructions into a whole variety of ways including, in particular, an in depth analysis and a wide variety of supervision from different modalities. I also encourage my students, psychotherapy supervisees and clients to put their mental and physical needs first.

Of course ta*king care of our selves* also requires a type of spiritual discipline. Sadly, the founders are now all dead, way before their time. In transactional analysis, we talk about life scripts, and, retrospectively, it does appear that they had tragic life scripts. I link this to the fact that they came from such a split and brutally unfair society in which they had been on the wrong side of goodness. They could not disguise from themselves that their privilege had been based on a system of the most virile racism ever to exist. I suspect their naturally moral temperaments meant that the toxicity of the system leaked into their very souls and hearts in unconscious ways, and maybe contributed in some ways to their early demise.

Driving to Metanoia

I had set the satellite navigation to drive to West London from West Sussex, a journey that should have taken about one and a half hours. The unconscious though has its own agenda, and instead of driving towards London I found myself driving towards Dover with the association of leaving on a ferry to go to France and beyond—away from the UK. I eventually pulled myself out of this deeply dissociative process and was able to shift into a more linear frame of mind.

I reflected on the fact that I was nervous about who I might meet in the group of 18 people who had elected to come to my course. My anxiety was linked to one of my last experiences at Metanoia when I had had a particularly nasty experience with a deeply misogynistic male trainee who was about to go on a placement to see female clients. I made a huge fuss about his inclusion on the course, which, at the time, ruptured some collegial relationships. Harmonious relationships had, however, since been established and the trainee in question had eventually been suspended.

The Group—Day One

I arrived 3 hours and 20 minutes after I had left my home. Fortunately, I had left plenty of time so was only 15 minutes late. I quickly ascertained which room I was to be teaching in. It was my favourite room in the institute, named Rogers after Carl Rogers. It was a beautiful large and airy room. As I walked in, I saw a group of what were clearly international participants. They were dressed in bright colours for the summer, and all, to my mind, seemed to be smiling a welcome to me. An immediate rapport emerged between us even as I hustled and bustled over to check the PowerPoint and then play hide and seek with my notes that seemed to be lost in my bag. We all began to giggle together as I made random noises and comments about my difficult journey, and where the hell were my notes. I could tell we were going to have fun in the best learning tradition I had learned in my own time as a trainee at Metanoia.

The Wailing Woman

The group included a rich collection of cultures, religions, and sexuality; including Arab, Jew, Hindu, and Secular; Asian, African, East European, American, Mexican, and Essex—one of the most working-class counties in the UK. It was a glorious opportunity to use the group's experience to teach transgenerational trauma. My teaching style is to start a conversation with group members as soon as they start to check in, making links with their checking in stories to the theme of transgenerational trauma. As we conversed, a Mexican woman shared the following story:

> Once a Spanish soldier married a beautiful native woman and they had two children whom the soldier loved very much. However, the soldier came from a rich family. His parents and relations disapproved of his wife and threatened to disown him unless he married a Spanish woman. Not wishing to lose his inheritance, the soldier put away his native wife and sent for a bride from Spain.

> The soldier's wife was filled with a terrible, jealous rage. To revenge herself against her unfaithful husband, she drowned their two children in the river. The soldier was horrified when he heard what she had done, and tried to have her arrested. But his wife, driven insane by rage, jealousy, and guilt, escaped into the wilds. She roamed through the land, searching the waterways for her children. But she could not find them. Finally, in agony of body and mind, she drowned herself in the river too.

But the woman's spirit could not escape to heaven because of the weight of her terrible crime. And so, La Llorona, the Wailing Woman, spirit still wanders the earth, wailing in guilt and grief. She is condemned forever to search in vain for her children. But she will never find them, for they are no more.

On listening to this story, I fell into a meditative state and began to tell them the story of Petruska's baby. I recalled how fairly early in my own training days, I had learned that Petruska had given birth to a baby who had later died in hospital. Members of the group were very interested to hear more about Petruska and I found myself telling them how sad I had always thought she was but that it had never been something I thought I could comment on. I described how Petruska had earned a prodigious reputation in the evolving British counselling and psychotherapy scene. Within Metanoia, she was admired and respected but this changed, for reasons I never fully understood, culminating in her loss of Metanoia as she turned against her former colleagues. I watched, along with others, feeling powerless, as Petruska lost yet another "baby"—Metanoia—in which she had invested so many of her dreams and desires. Her downward spiral after this loss appeared inevitable; it was as if she was repeating loss over and over—maybe. Who knows. The group were aghast to hear that she had committed suicide and, as I told them the story of Petruska's final act on this earth, I felt again the shock of it. Since the theme was transgenerational trauma, we reflected on the traumatic history she had inherited and how the privilege she had been part of had also been a poisoned chalice. I was also thoughtful about how little the students knew of their organisation's history which wasn't that old and yet it was as if it was kept hidden in some way, not as a conscious act but as a type of unconscious enactment maybe.

However this conversation captured the group's imagination. They were open and expressive about their own experiences. Many stories emerged of lost babies, grieving mothers, and traumas passed on through generations, setting the emotional agenda for the weekend's teaching.

The Group—Day Two

The next morning we began as we had left off, as though the conversation had simply had a semi-colon after the last words. "I googled Petruska Clarkson last night," began a quietly spoken member of the group. "Did you know that today is the anniversary of her death?"

A silence descended on the room. I had not known that this was the date; and yet, maybe I had. I just did not know that I knew until now, reminiscent of unthought knowns (Bollas, 1987). I have thought about this process often since that weekend.

Reflections on This Process

Shortly after being asked to write this article, I received a copy of *Psychoanalytic Dialogues* in which there was an article entitled "Becoming a Telepathic Tuning Fork" by Sharon K. Farber (2017).

Tony Bass (2001) quotes Farber making links with this type of unconscious interconnectedness.

Tony Bass in his article supports her ideas of the "tundig fork" which I relate to. I am familiar with many of her references and conceptual language, which she draws on to make the case for telephathic connection.

When did the process actually begin? In telling the story of Petruska, I recalled my receptivity to the state of her mind many years earlier. Her sadness had impressed itself upon me more than any other thing about her, although I never actually talked about it with anyone. This type of receptivity tends to eclipse ordinary linear thought and has been a strong characteristic of mine, even as a child. This could also be understood as a type of dissociative process between me and Petruska in which her disavowed sadness communicated with my dissociated sadness (I had lost two babies in utero). Perhaps this dissociative process was awakened by the student who told the story of the Wailing Woman. Maybe the student's attuned unconscious receptivity awakened something in me that made it possible for

> a form of human experience not quite like any other, through sharing elements in common with other relationships of intense resonance, intimacy, car, vulnerability, and mutual personal and interpersonal knowledge.
>
> (Bass, 2001, p. 701)

Maybe my attempt to "escape the country" was an attempt to avoid the anniversary which I did not know about, but did know. When Petruska killed herself, I fell into a deep depression and never fully understood it. Now I wonder if it was linked to this sense that the loss of her "babies" was intolerable; that the loss of my unborn babies was also, somehow, intolerable. Farber quotes Bass who posed a question related to quantum physics, which connects everything in the universe (an idea that Petruska often promoted in her own teachings).

> Could it be that we have discovered or created a form of human relatedness in which … a connection so profound wrought is never truly broken, irrespective of apparent distances of time and space.
>
> (Bass, 2001 cited by Farber 2017, p. 701)

Synchronicity, according to Jung, is when events that appear to just be coincidence are actually pregnant with meaning. This event seemed to me to be synchronous. Was there even a telepathic communication from Petruska, from the "other side," wanting her story to be heard, her loss validated? Was she still out there somewhere, looking in the rivers for her abandoned babies? Was she returning to reclaim her rightful place at Metanoia? Whatever the rights and wrongs of what had happened to her, there is no doubt that without Petruska there would be no Metanoia Institute, no group, no Options weekend, no course, no me, no them, no us! She gave birth to us; but that had somehow got lost in the ensuing years. How was it that the group knew nothing, or very little, about the founding Mother of the organisation? Was it through me, she was returning? Perhaps, in some grandiose way, I like to think that is the case. I too had "lost" Metanoia, and now was returning with "something" that was trying to make itself conscious through me. Maybe I knew this somewhere and had been trying to avoid it—escape to France! "Telepathy can be understood as a type of unconscious affective communication or implicit relational knowing" (Stern et al 1998 cited in Farber 2017, p. 723). It is not just about me though. What about the group process? For instance, was the unconscious making itself heard through the story of the Wailing Woman told by the student from Mexico? Were we all involved in a type of group projective identification? As Bass (2001, asks in his article entitled, "It Takes One to Know One, or, Whose Unconscious Is.

Political Analysis and the Theory of Trans Generational Trauma: The Personal is Political—How the Past Informs the Present

The most recent research and paradigm shift in psychoanalysis/psycho-therapy is in the area of transgenerational trauma. Trauma is an event that has not been experienced, strangely enough, but occupies a part of our psyche, often in the format of deadness, nothingness, and emptiness. When mourning is avoided and repressed (Freud 1917; Gerson 2009; Green 2001; Leader 2009), the melancholic fugue that descends upon the victim keeps them (and us?) from feeling truly alive. This process is highly contagious and can take over a group's consciousness. Winnicott (1984) describes the sub-lime beauty and purity of the "maternal gaze." He did tend to idolise the maternal and, partly, this may have been because he was sent away early to public school. Nevertheless, there is such a gaze. But what if the gaze that is reflected back to the infant is contaminated with brokenness and grief? What then is ingested and introjected with the mother's milk?

In the emerging theory of epigenetics, scientists have discovered that trauma is coded in the body in terms of cortisol levels and receptor site alterations (Yehuda 2014). Trauma changes the person's body and mind, and then their children are pre-disposed bodily and psychically to being raised by these traumatised parents. Research shows that a traumatic trigger in the present, often "activates" transgenerational trauma. These ghosts, unmetabolised trauma, remain in the embryo. It is conceivable that those of us drawn to examine our lives, because of personal suffering, have perhaps found it incumbent upon us to be the "chosen ones"—those who are required by some type of cosmic law to metabolise the trauma. Within transactional analysis , Fanita English (1969) referred to this process as passing the "hot potato" down through the generations. I have found it rewarding to work with groups of people from diverse backgrounds because it makes the group process richer as we all engage with the various ways in which our people, who have suffered in the past, have found their way into the present. This divergence of traumatic experience makes it possible to deepen and enrich a more collective understanding of loss and trauma. Often this requires witnessing and validating experiences from the past so they become real.

Over the years, I have found it necessary to have conversations about religion, powerful organisations, wars, famines, the holocaust, colonisation, slavery, and family abusive situations. When participants of the group share knowledge and relational stories about such events, this in itself constitutes a metabolisation of various traumas. The process of meaning-making is healing for all of us and our clients. Everyone's mind is particularly enriched (in a non linear way) through a profound experience of meaning making that is then taken back into the clinical situation—not as an instruction, but more as an internalised experience which implicitly informs the clinical situation.

In Conclusion—Living Symbolically (Jung, 1978)

As psychotherapists, we are required to engage in the world of symbols, of meaning making. When we are open to this process, it becomes more natural to observe how much more satisfying it is to find meaning in our lives in non linear ways. Psychotherapy, at it most potent, helps the right brain expand and supports the integration of dissociated "not me" states. The members of the group chose to attend a workshop on transgenerational trauma for diverse reasons. The ensuing alchemy we co created was, I believe, on some level, transformative for us all. At the time many approached me for therapy and supervision to which I could not respond; but now, I think it was in an effort to continue a conversation that they now needed to do in their own analysis.

REFLECTIONS

The impetus for this article is clearly expressed in the description of how the weekend unfolded. The article speaks for itself. I think it is testimony to how the right hemisphere of our brains communicate with each other. "The newer fields of affective neuroscience and especially social neuroscience are exploring inter-brain interactions" (Schore. 2003ap. 214).

This session at metanoia was, without doubt, the most unusual experience I have ever had as a tutor. As a group, we seemed to co create a bond of emotional and psychological attachment from the very beginning. Perhaps it was even before the beginning as I drove frantically through Southern England going further and further from my destination. Maybe I was trying to avoid "something" while the group waited patiently and expectantly. Were we already in communication with each other? On some level, it felt to me that I was in an infant self-state, coming in from my circuitous journey to be welcomed by nurturing parental self states? When I experienced their welcome with gratitude and recognition, we seemed to form a union through which so many experiences revealed themselves. Mystical and magical! Not words we tend to pay attention to in our profession and yet, as the scientists tell us, we only really understand 5% of the universe so what hope for what we can understand of the psyche!

Chapter 7

Anna Karenina, Lilly, and the Co-created Unconscious Relational Third

Helena Hargaden

"The principle method of co-creative transactional analysis is best considered as a generative approach" (Summers, 2014, p. xxxvii). In this chapter, I introduce the idea of the "third," a concept which, I propose, has the potential to expand and enrich the theoretical range of co-creative transactional analysis. In the following case study, I demonstrate how the "third" is generated by the cocreated relational unconscious and facilitates "the emergence of new contextually viable possibilities grounded in relational experience" (ibid., xxxvii).

When invited to write this contribution, I thought of "Lilly" because of what happened between us about which I say more later. The "third" refers to the creation of a triangular space, alongside the therapist and client, that enables the therapy to move beyond an impasse in the dyadic relationship, and "allows for more nuanced and 'mature' forms of relating to both self and others" (Gerson, 2006 posting). The original idea of the "third" derives from an understanding of how the "father"-father is a metaphor that stands for any other person or object such as the mother's work for instance-interrupts the Oedipal process so that mother and child are separated by a "third" other, enabling the child to move out of the symbiotic relationship with mother. In the therapeutic relationship, the "third" is characterised by many things, one of which could be the therapist's thoughts, which may be experienced as an intrusion into the empathic flow of the therapeutic relationship. Gerson (2004) suggests three categories of potential thirds: developmental, cultural, and relational. Developmental thirdness acknowledges the third position as an Oedipal constellation and is represented in the work of Britton (1998); the cultural third is one which envelops and shapes the interactions of the dyad and is represented by the work of Chasseguet-Smirgel (1974) and Lacan (1977); the relational third is most frequently associated with an intersubjective perspective, as developed in the work of Bollas (1987), Ogden (2004), Benjamin (2004), and Orange (1997). My focus here is on the relational "third," the emergence of which changed the course of the therapy in the following account.

DOI: 10.4324/9781032266237-8

When Lilly first walked into my consulting room, I did not see a 30-year-old woman. From the way she moved, her childish dress, her hair in bobbins, I saw, instead, a child: demure, pretty, and dainty. Her name is of course not Lilly, that is my name for her, and there must be some meaning in that. Lilly is the name of a flower that is pretty, fragrant, elegant, and a mark of culture. There is "something else," though, about the name for I found myself humming a folk song called "Lilly of the West," which is the name given to a woman who betrays her lover by falling in love with another man. Lilly's rejection turns him into a killer and yet, despite being sentenced, he still loves his "faithless" Lilly of the West. My association with this folk song reveals the shadow side of "Lilly," which makes her more interesting, opening up a secret domain of a woman who has sexual power and independence of mind.

The thoughts of Lilly as a powerful, sexual, independent, although "faithless" young woman, if they existed at all, were remote from my conscious mind as I embarked on my work with Lilly. I experienced her as childlike, unnecessarily adapted to others' needs and emotionally hidden. It turned out that Lilly was no stranger to therapy, having been in classical transactional analysis, which seemed to reinforce her belief that there was something pathological about her feelings, which she defined as rackets. This made it impossible to get close to her as she described herself and her feelings in such concrete and derogatory terms. When telling her story she showed little affect: her father had left her mother when Lilly was twelve; her mother was devastated and had gone into a depressed fugue. The family's circumstance deteriorated, and Lilly lost the security of home and parents. Lilly seemed to have no feelings about any of this. Both parents sounded self-absorbed as, too, was her new stepmother, for whom Lilly felt obliged to be the "cute" and loving object.

The atmosphere that emerged between us in the relationship was one of me feeling irritable, sometimes angry, even enraged as Lilly smiled and twinkled her way through the sessions. In her current life, she was in an unsatisfactory relationship with a man whom she felt she must placate, and around whom she had to be cute, and "supportive" of his needs, dreams, and requests of her with little thought of her own ambitions and needs. It was confusing to me that she was clearly well-educated and articulate, and even held down an important job for a prestigious organisation, yet Lilly felt to me like a girl, who experienced herself as quite powerless, and whose main function was to play supportive roles to others in her life, and to be whatever they needed her to be. Stuck in a crippling paralysis of internalised symbiotic relationships, Lilly felt required to be compliant, adapted and to repress her true experiences.

The co-created dynamic that ensued involved me in "chasing" Lilly with my thoughts and, although I introduced my countertransference reflectively, and Lilly did make some changes, there was a deep reluctance on her part to let me really know her. She resisted my curiosity, for instance, about her work, and any of my attempts to relate to her as a powerful adult woman. The therapy felt polarised into a parent-child configuration.

The incident that altered this dynamic was the emergence of the co-created "third" between us in the form of the book, *Anna Karenina*, by Leo Tolstoy (1877/2000).

A few weeks before my summer break, Lilly arrived for her session looking even more child-like than usual in a floral pinafore dress and white socks. As she sat down, she smilingly told me that, as she had walked up the hill to my house, she had been reading her book and a man had behaved inappropriately towards her. I was infuriated, as though with a daughter who had put herself in danger. I shared my thoughts rather more forcefully than usual and Lilly felt hurt and angry with me, feeling criticised and blamed for attracting unwelcome male attention. Unusually, over the following weeks, she expressed her anger with me; she thought I had been too harsh with her, and she felt hurt by me. We talked about the situation at length in a way which felt as though the roles had been reversed: I was the Child and she was the Parent, telling me off for being impatient with her and saying "horrible" things. We were stuck in an impasse, when, on the last day before my holiday, I found myself, slightly impatiently, cutting across the repetitive dialogue with a question: "What were you reading anyway?" "Anna Karenina" she replied. In that moment, I saw Lilly afresh: who was she? I was curious.

So, on holiday, I read the book. In it Tolstoy describes a society, which is obsessed with status, image, material gain, easy pleasures gained through gambling, sex, intrigues, mindless projects, and a narcissistic community full of its own self-importance. Anna, although fascinating and wonderfully seductive, is essentially self-absorbed, amoral, and self-pitying. Levin, an anti-hero, on the periphery of the "in" crowd to which Anna belongs, turns out to be the unlikely, but real hero of the story. At the beginning of the book, he seems boorish, moralistic, too serious, and unpopular but, unlike Anna, he is willing to struggle with himself, to engage honestly with his frustration. By the end of the book, he finds how to live a satisfying life whilst Anna is destroyed by her narcissism.

I found the book deeply satisfying and was grateful to Lilly for re-introducing me to Tolstoy. Lilly was very surprised when I told her that I had read the book and shocked to hear that I was interested in her views about the characters and what she thought about the moral tone of the book. Her reflections on the themes, including the fantasy of narcissistic love, and the reality of love led to her musing on what really mattered to her, on what she wanted from life. The emergence of this "third" into our work provided Lilly with a language to discover domains of herself that had hitherto been hidden. This "third" enabled us to move beyond our individual psyches, and a stale impasse, into here and now Adult–Adult relatedness.

Thirdness, as Gerson (2006) described it, is: "that quality of human existence that transcends individuality, permits and constricts that which can be known, and wraps all of our sensibilities in ways that we experience as simultaneously alien as well as part of ourselves." (p. 66). The "third" allowed the therapy to become more vital when it had previously suffered from elements of deadness, to evolve, take on a more improvised feel; it became more possible to play around with ideas. As Summers puts it his introduction: "The principle method of co-creative transactional analysis is play" (p. xxxvii).

Our reflections helped Lilly to disentangle from the crucifying symbiotic relations. She became more conscious of her stuckness and the rage she felt with her parents. This acknowledgement by her enabled her to become more autonomous. There is of course so much more to say about Lilly. The major focus of this case however is to illustrate an understanding of how the "third" can bring about a more co-created dynamic within transactional analysis.

REFLECTIONS

Although I consciously experienced my client as driving me "mad" with irritation, especially when she referred to reading Anna Karenina on her way to see me as described in the chapter, I now realise that the very source of our rupture, was also the rich source of our repair.

In his article, the "dead third" (Gerson, 2009) describes how something as calamitous as the holocaust resides as a type of dead third in the mind. In this client's case, there was nothing so obviously traumatic but her deadness pointed to a different type of trauma—one where there exists a type of lacuna. This deadness was brought alive by the richness and complexity of Anna Karenina. Tolstoy brought life into a therapy that was overwhelmingly boring until we had conversations that went on for months about Anna. I found a rich source of intelligence and active imagination that had previously seemed impossible. Thank you Mr. Tolstoy!

Chapter 8

Remember, Remember, the Fifth of November

Helena Hargaden

Remember, remember,
the fifth of November,
Gunpowder, treason and plot.
We see no reason why
Gunpowder treason
Should ever be forgot.
> (Nursery rhyme about Guy Fwkes Night, celebrated in Britain on
> 5 November with fireworks, bonfires, and effigy burning to commem-
> orate the 1605 "Gunpowder Plot" to blow up the English Parliament
> along with King James I in hopes of sparking an uprising of English
> Catholics over severe laws against the practice of their religion.)

It was dark and cold; it was that time of year, again. The clocks had gone back the previous week and though it was now completely dark, I had forgotten to close the curtains. Maya sat opposite me, trembling with fear and jumping at every sound. I was not quite calm myself, for the cacophony of noise outside was, at times, deafening. Each year, with unfailing and, to my mind, depressing regularity, the noise of the thunderous Guy Fawkes fireworks shrieking through the November air intruded on the environment.

Maya seemed unusually perturbed this night. I recalled her words from the same time last year: "I am terrified, I hate them." On inquiry, it seemed that the noise must have echoed somewhere in her unconscious from her days as a toddler, in the Second World War; hiding under the stairs from the falling bombs, she recalled only a sense of aloneness and feelings of terror. I looked at her now, feeling helpless. Nothing in the last year had apparently changed, and I was at a loss as to how to access these feelings and experiences and how, in some way, to facilitate a metabolisation or transformation of the terror that so often seemed to be subsumed by a type of paralysis between us. Of course, we had talked and tried to make sense of what it

DOI: 10.4324/9781032266237-9

would have been like for the child hiding under the stairs. We had both "felt" for her, but we were both left with a sense of futility about how to help and a sense of the artificiality of trying to conjure up the scene.

Some weeks later, we were again sitting opposite each other and sensing paralysis in the therapy, a type of frozenness between us—not that there were hard feelings, just that it was hard to access any feelings except anxiety. I recalled how when I first met Maya, I thought there was something hardened, not fluid, not accessible about her; and although I came to like her and appreciate her intelligence, I sometimes experienced her as rather cold and unaffected by serious upsets that had happened in her life. No amount of cognitive transacting could change this, and I often felt frustrated with the sense of paralysis in our relationship.

An idea began to formulate in my mind. As I sat feeling my "not feeling," I felt my presence as a type of obstacle to something, and it occurred to me that Maya needed to lie down on the couch. I had been on the couch in my own Jungian analysis for several years, so I did not feel that it was too strange a suggestion. In fact, the idea occurred to me with a type of urgency, that this was precisely what Maya needed. I was unsure how she might take it since I had never even indicated that it was a possibility; but I need not have worried. Maya seemed immediately to see the suggestion as a creative opportunity for something different to occur, and so we began a prolonged period (about 18 months) with Maya on the couch.

As soon as she lay down, Maya entered a type of dream world and began to engage with a stream of dark, negative, frightening images involving a small figure embarked on a terrifying journey through a dismal and bleak landscape. There were often winding paths, overgrown fields, dark and empty buildings, witches hats, threatening creatures, and dangerous looking machines. Pervasive themes included isolation, despair, bleakness, and threat. After each therapy hour, Maya returned home and painted, and each week she brought a new painting to her session. They represented her dream world from the previous week. We looked at them together, and I commented vaguely on what I saw, although intuitively I felt it would be unhelpful to say too much. Maya had embarked on a journey that seemed to have its own momentum and raison d'etre, and I participated as a type of benign, attentive, thoughtful, but essentially nonintrusive presence. I wondered what we were doing and how it was going, but I trusted that we would find out as we went along.

I knew this did not sound like TA, but that is what I trained in. So what was I doing? I could account for the use of the couch as putting Maya in more direct contact with her Child ego state and her unconscious. And her inner landscape was consistent with Berne's (1961) descriptions of primal images, intuitions, fairy tales, and the transference drama. Nevertheless, over the years I had come to recognise that despite my struggle to stay true to traditional TA, I had failed miserably. My clinical experience had taught me that I needed to develop my thinking and methodology. Indeed, my clients taught me how to change the theory; and, as a result, my colleague Charlotte Sills and I (Hargaden & Sills, 2002) developed a relational theory of TA.

In particular, Charlotte and I concentrated on a model of transferential domains that allows for multiple ways of relating with concomitant multiple technical choices. This model is based on the idea that transference is ubiquitous in life as well as in therapy, and that there are three distinct types of transference: introjective, projective, and transformational. These are not necessarily discreet and may overlap and be interconnected. In essence, the model returns to the psychoanalytic roots of TA while retaining and developing the notion of transactions between therapist and client. Our model thus acts as a conceptual bridge between intrapsychic processes and the relationship between therapist and client. In my work with Maya, for example, I no longer had to remain within a narrow framework of what was considered TA. With the relational TA model, I had a variety of choices with regard to technique, intervention, and treatment direction.

One important effect of the model is that it allows for deeper engagement with the unconscious. With Maya, the time on the couch gave evidence of this unconscious processing, and my way of working with her can best be described as working within the introjective transference. This form of transference allows for the creation of a container in which both therapist and client appear to fence off elements of reality while "something" else happens. P. Casement (personal communication, November 2002) described this as the "required relationship." In this transferential domain, the therapist needs to become a type of Echo; but a conscious, rather than an adapted or needy, one, as described in the myth of Narcissus. The therapist's job is to hold the tension between the pressure and demands from the client to reflect a perfect mirror of their persona, while looking for opportunities to "echo" the often distant and subtle strains of feelings emanating from the heart and soul of the unknown or deeply repressed sense of self.

It has now been well established by neurological findings that emotion operates as a central organising process within the brain, that the emotional quality of early attachments influences an individual's ability to engage with and integrate experiences. This suggests that the evolving emotional sense of self will be the key to unlocking the client's true sense of self-love and worth. Thus, within the introjective transference, as the client uses the therapist as an emotional container who emotionally mirrors them, they are able to introject an emotional sense of self, as though they were part of the therapist rather than a separate being.

Maya was a fairly conservative woman, socially very skilled. The only way to unlock her Child, it seemed to me, was to remove myself—the Other to whom she needed to comply, be sociable, and be nice—from the situation by her going on the couch. In this way, I provided an emotional ambience without intruding my "self" into the relationship during this phase.

As well as an individual session, Maya also attended group once a week. There we engaged at a more openly relational level as the format seemed to release her ability to be angry with me. She felt I did not pay her enough attention, that she was insignificant and did not matter. She felt silenced by me and sometimes dismissed or made fun of. I looked to my own behaviour and, when it was the case, I acknowledged the truth. But I also refused to conform to her needs to be made special. At the same time, I consciously stroked her for her achievements, in particular, the abilities she revealed in making a warm, convivial home for herself and her relatives and the talent she showed for engaging in fun relationships with her grandchildren. I was mindful that some of the dynamics described in her stream of consciousness, and sometimes enacted with me, replicated her relationship with her mother, who sounded seriously preoccupied with her own life and barely conscious of her daughter's existence or needs. In the group, Maya seemed able to project some of her introjected vicious Parent and conjoined angry Child ego states onto me and work them through. Charlotte Sills and I refer to this process as the projective transference, one in which the therapist is actively engaged in interpreting, illustrating, and confronting (Berne, 1966/1994). The countertransference with projective transference is more active and alive, whereas the countertransference with introjective transference requires a more concentrated type of focus on the emerging Child ego states.

The third domain of transference—transformation transference—is one in which unthought, unmetabolised, and primitive experience becomes transformed. Maya's time on the couch reflected this process. Transformational transference is most similar to projective identification in that there is an unconscious relationship between therapist and client. We could say that this unconscious relatedness was reflected in my unusual decision to suggest the couch to Maya. Although a conservative person, she immediately agreed to it, almost as though she had suggested it. The pressure I felt when sitting opposite her to somehow remove myself had perhaps emanated from her in the first place—a communication from her unconscious to my unconscious that resulted in my behaving in ways I normally do not behave. This is a strong feature of projective identification and one that allows for processing experiences that are unconscious but lodged in some traumatic way within the client's psyche.

From the perspective of relational TA, the process with Maya could be understood to involve work in all three transferential domains. The projective one predominated in group; whereas in individual sessions, we were in the introjective and transformational domains most of the time, with me as an attentive, nonintrusive, emotionally responsive person with no subjective life of my own—yet actively drawn into engaging with primitive and terrifying experiences. Both situations laid the foundation for us to move into a more intersubjective relationship, one in which both of our subjectivities could coexist (Hargaden & Fenton, 2005).

One day, Maya stopped lying on the couch. We did not really discuss it. She no longer felt the need and neither did I. We were now able, it seemed, to sit opposite each other without the dreadful sense of paralysis; instead, a sense of closeness began to emerge. We had been through a long, difficult journey together, and at that point, we seemed to embark on a new relationship in which Maya could confide in me more easily, be less controlled with me and less controlling of me, and I began to feel a real sense of her warmth and softness.

Relational TA is concerned with interactions in which the whole person of the therapist—their subjectivity—is fundamentally implicated in the therapeutic encounter and the process of change (Cornell & Hargaden, 2005). In the therapy with Maya, it is clear how my subjectivity was engaged at every turn, but in a variety of ways. My reflections were largely intuitive; yet on deeper inquiry, I can recognise significant aspects of who I am that influenced the work with Maya. Not the least of these, of course, was the time I spent on the couch with an echoing presence behind me, most often experienced as a loving acceptance of my rambling thoughts and emerging unthought-through feeling states, states that eventually came to feel a part of who I now am.

It was November again. I noticed I had forgotten to close the curtains, and the dark night yawned out in front of us through the windows. A screaming shriek of fireworks burst into the darkness. I jumped. Maya blinked several times, but not in fear—more in the way one might flick off an irritating mosquito. She was in full flight and her face was animated not by fear, but by sexual desire. She had met a man and she was keen, "but just for sex," she said. I thought, "hmm, I don't think it's just for sex," but then that might be me and the promptings of my now distant Catholic childhood. Eventually sex did feature hugely and wonderfully in their relationship, and indeed in ours. It brought us together like mother and daughter, bride and bridesmaid, friends giggling confidentially over well-kept secrets. Such was the warmth between us now that I could barely imagine how I had ever thought of Maya as cold or hard; it did not seem possible. It seemed that the terrifying images that had hidden behind her paralysis were now converted into energy that was, to my delighted surprise, deeply sexual.

It is November yet again. Maya is leaving in December to travel around the world with her new husband. She does not mention fireworks, and I find myself feeling calmed by her composure as the fireworks scream and shriek their way through the skies. This time I have remembered to close the curtains, and we feel snug, warm, and cosy wrapped up in our closeness. But this belies the truth of the situation, for we are about to part, and it is hard. Sometimes Maya tries to get rid of me rather quickly and "move on," as she puts it. Other times we struggle to find words to describe our experience together. I, too, at times, withdraw and feel distant. I do not like goodbyes, and sometimes it feels too hard to be a psychotherapist. Another firework screams through the skies, and I think that Guy Fawkes night will never seem quite the same to me again.

REFLECTIONS

This was a short piece I wrote for the ITA (Institute of Transactional Analysis) News. I worked with this client in a way, which differed from my usual face to face meetings. In our initial meetings, I felt that we could not move beyond her politeness, her need to get it "right," to assure me of her "goodness." I was on the couch in my own Jungian analysis; and although I did not require all of my clients to go on the couch, sometimes it just felt necessary as it did with this client. My intuition was accurate. Once on the couch, she travelled on a journey that was full of images, terrifying, full of noise, thuds, banging that was mirrored each year bonfire night in the UK. This client found it difficult to access feelings but she found her way through art, which expressed the terror she could not articulate. Because it involved her experience as a child in the Second World War, I thought it would interest those readers of the ITA News who came from a similar generation to her. I thought the symbolic meaning she arrived at through her art would generate recognition for others of what they may have also experienced.

Damasio (1999) describes how the neurological evidence simply suggests that selective absence of emotion is a problem. Well-tried and well-deployed emotion seems to be a support system without which the edifice of reason cannot operate properly. It was through her art that she enabled me to contact my feelings, as previously I had found it hard to connect with her since she was very rational and cognitive in her narrative telling. It was through her art that I was eventually able to identify the feelings deeply buried and in this way found closeness, connection, and intimacy. She could not sustain this in the group because it was too vulnerable and potentially shaming. I contact my feelings directly and am not a person who connects with art so easily, as she did, but our way of working together enabled us to meet and connect.

The story of Guy Fawkes is a compelling story of loss, betrayal, hatred, love, insurrection, fire, and terror. It was that story and the actual event that influenced our connection. We both related to the story but from very different perspectives. Yet, the story brought us together. I could get her sense of terror. I could hate the fireworks as vividly as she did but for different reasons. When she eventually worked through this, she no longer bothered so much about the fireworks, and I, too, found my anxiety and terror lessened as I listened to her plans for marriage. When I think about this therapy now, I feel grateful and loving toward her—for she changed me as much as I changed her. Nothing changes if the therapist doesn't change!

Chapter 9

Building Resilience
The Role of Firm Boundaries and the Third in Relational Group Therapy

Helena Hargaden

Richard Erskine's (2013) article "Relational Group Process: Developments in a Transactional Analysis Model of Group Psychotherapy" gives an elegant and informative account of his clinical evolution as a group psychotherapist. I found much to agree with in his approach to relational group process, for example, in his critique of the feedback model he speaks for many of us who have learned, through experience, that direct confrontation in groups can feel overwhelming and shaming and can be clinically ineffective. I resonate entirely with his aim for group therapy to be "coconstructive and relational, that is truly indigenous to the group" (p. 165/262).

In response to Erskine, I want to examine the importance he places on safety and empathic, respectful contact in group therapy. I suggest a different way of focusing on these factors by proposing a model of group therapy that allows for the emergence of aggression in group dynamics while avoiding destruction of the group.

Empathy

The therapeutic role of empathy is indisputable according to the research (Asay & Lambert, 1999). Empathy, although not without a feeling component, is essentially a cognitive function that the therapist uses to let the client know he or she has understood what the person is saying and feeling. (Sometimes this happens even if the therapist does not understand but can make it appear that he or she does.) Empathy is mostly an intellectual performance, albeit an extremely useful method to oil the wheels of the therapeutic alliance—or misalliance depending on what else happens in the therapy.

While there is, undoubtedly, a place for empathy in a group, if all group members must be carefully considerate of one another, where is the space for other, more primitive feelings to emerge? Although in his article, Erskine recognises that an overuse of empathy can produce "niceness," I do not think he goes far enough in his critique to analyse the potentially negative impact of empathy or what I refer to as the *shadow* side of empathy. This refers to unconscious aspects that are not recognised by the conscious self.

DOI: 10.4324/9781032266237-10

In the case of empathy, for example, it seems, at first glance, to be a good thing. However, Guggenbuhl-Craig (1971) suggested that empathy can be used to bind the patient more firmly to the therapist since, in the patient's eyes, the therapist "has become someone who apparently sees the greatest value in something which might not appear so very valuable at first glance" (p. 73). In other words, the use of empathy can endow a false sense of self-esteem that I believe interferes with the development of resilience.

In a different but equally important critique, Hoffman (1992) asserted that empathy may be experienced by the client as a self-protective strategy by which the therapist is hiding some aspect of himself or herself. This critique is important for group therapy situations in which members can use empathy as a mask and defense against being discovered or seen or discovering and seeing. By striving to behave empathically, there is the danger of the group becoming the idealised mother who understands perfectly, making it seem that everything can be understood.

Attunement

I agree with Erskine (2013) when he describes attunement as a process of being "with others' inner experience, a resonance with their affect" (p. 268), but when he continues that it is also about tuning in to their "self-perspective, and how they make meaning" (p. 267) he is implying conscious intent. A central feature of attunement, however, is that it is a nonconscious process involving deep feeling processes (countertransference) in which meaning only comes retrospectively. For example, the therapist and other group members may attune to an unconscious affect that will not be immediately recognised by the other and may differ from his or her self-perspective. This especially seems to be the case with aggression, when the person's self-perspective is at odds with a self that feels threatening to his or her conscious view of himself or herself. Beebe and Lachmann (1992) described attunement when they observed how infants, in mutually affective relationships with caretakers, moved in and out of synchronicity, contact, ruptures, and repairs. They described these nonverbal engagements as protoconversations that are made up of gesture, rhythm, and musicality. The term "musicality" might falsely lead to the conclusion that attunement involves an all-loving, warm feeling, but one only has to think of the nervous anticipation induced by Beethoven's Fifth Symphony, for example, to reconsider the meaning. All parents who have raised babies know how easy it is to be induced into a state of rage and terror by the infant and the emotional challenge of containing and processing these primitive feelings. Attunement will, therefore, be the more likely route that sets the group on a path of struggle and by which primitive feelings will be expressed and tuned in to. Attunement is the vehicle by which subjectivities that have previously been unknown can emerge into consciousness. In a group, members may find themselves unconsciously attuning to the body position of others, unexpectedly feeling tears well up or righteous anger swelling, noticing a deep-seated sigh escaping from their lips, or experiencing a somatic response such as a stomach ache or itching. These are not cognitive responses but are based on an evolving nonverbal conversation. These attuned experiences provide the unconscious template for enactments.

The Beginning of an Enactment in Group Therapy

In a monologue, Yvonne yells at the therapist, outlining the therapist's faults as she sees them. Stunned into silence by the ferocity of the attack, the therapist freezes inside; she cannot find her mind (Bion, 1959). But in a tiny corner of her mind, she is able to hold onto the thought that she must not react. I shall call this tiny corner of her mind the *third*. With this term, I am referring to an interruption into the dyadic relationship, about which I will say more later.

The Role of Safety in Group Therapy

While I agree with Erskine that safety is important in groups, I think that the location of such safety is in the boundary, not the interpersonal contact. The type of interpersonal carefulness suggested by Erskine invites a faux sense of connection, closing down the opportunity for enactment of disturbed experience as group participants try to find empathic and considerate ways to avoid aggression. An enactment involves acting out experiences that are simultaneously impossible to forget and impossible to tell. The evidence is clear that enactments are not only inevitable but create opportunities for insight, metabolisation, and even transformation (Frawley-O'Dea, 1997; Gabbard, 1992; Hargaden, 2010).

Because relational therapy involves an excavation of unconscious processes, safety needs to be located primarily in the provision of firm boundaries. Jung (1978) introduced the metaphor of the *alchemical container* in an attempt to capture the mystery, significance, and essence of the type of containment required if the unconscious is going to be able to do the work of healing. Continuing with the metaphor of alchemy, in the case of group therapy, it is the therapist and group who cocreate the container in which elements/processes are trapped. For release and transformation to occur, the container must be protected while the processes (transferences) mutate, turning the *nigredo* (dark materials brought in by the unconscious) into gold (the discovery of self). This is why, when group members understandably wish to make the group into a social one, or want to make contact with each other outside of group meetings in the mistaken belief that they will continue to find it as satisfying, it is up to the therapist to hold the boundary and not allow the intrusion of external thirds (this term is expanded on later) that would alter the potential for real change to take place. It needs to be reiterated that sexual boundaries between group members and obviously the therapist need to be clear and unequivocal. It is the firmness of these boundaries and the therapist's strength and ethical commitment to protecting them that makes the group a safe place. Within the boundaries, it then becomes possible for anything to be said, thus making it more likely that the darkest thoughts and feelings can be enacted and aired. Group members know that such thoughts and feelings will never be used against anyone, interpreted in a social setting, or used to seduce, manipulate, or exploit each other financially, sexually, or interpersonally. It is only in such a sealed container that it is safe to go through the enactments required for mental growth.

The Role of the Group Leader in the Development of Group Culture

Group members will take their lead based on their unconscious and intuitive sense of the leader's psychological state. It follows that the type of group culture that evolves will depend on the extent to which the therapist has engaged with his or her own early traumas and understands the potential for unconscious reenactment of his or her painful experiences, narcissistic needs to avoid conflict, and desire to be seen as good. The group will sense the therapist's emotional resilience in the way he or she establishes himself or herself as a group leader. In this way of working with relational processes, one of the main tasks for the therapist is to initiate the cocreation of a psychological space in which it is understood that enactments will occur; that group members will feel disturbed, unsettled, at times even frightened; that there is nothing that cannot be thought about or spoken about; and that meaning comes from reflecting on such experiences.

Using the Third to Think About Safety in Relational Group Dynamics

I agree with Erskine that it is important to create an environment of qualitative listening and reflection, but I propose a different way of creating it. The reason the method is different is because in this way of working, group members will be less careful and considered in what they express. There is, therefore, huge potential for blaming and shame, especially after an enactment. How then is it possible to restore the equilibrium provided by reflective listening in such a situation?

One way is the use of what I described earlier as the third. This refers to the creation of a triangular space, alongside the therapist and client, that enables the therapy to move beyond an impasse in the dyadic relationship. It paves the way for more subtle and discriminating forms of relating to both self and others. There are many potential thirds. Gerson (2004) divided them into three categories: developmental, relational, and cultural.

The Developmental Third

The original idea of the third derives from an understanding of how the "father" interrupts the dyadic relationship between the mother and child ("father" is a metaphor for any person or object, such as the mother's work, a grandparent, or a same-sex partner). In this configuration, the father provides a third in the relationship, separating mother and child and enabling the movement out of symbiosis. In the therapeutic relationship, the third can be characterised by many things, one of which is the therapist's thoughts if they are experienced as an intrusion into the empathic flow of the therapeutic relationship. An example is one of his patients telling Ron Britton (1989) to "stop that fucking thinking!" (p. 88).

The Cultural Third

The cultural third refers to the cultural contexts in which our subjectivities are shaped, including linguistic structures that influence how we think and feel. An obvious example is the use of language in the UK, where there are many different dialects, and nuances and forms of expression differ widely. For instance, what might be considered rude or mocking in a middle-class London suburb might have the connotation of friendliness and comradeship in a northern town such as Liverpool. An example of intercontinental difference is when an Indian woman in a group appeared to be governed by more sexist cultural expectations than did Western women in the group. On the other hand, she portrayed a powerful personality through her use of direct language, owning her power with a passion that illuminated the more timid expression of subjectivity observed in her apparently more liberated sisters.

The Relational Third

The relational third refers to an innate sense of self with other that we bring to every meeting with another. Ogden (2004) extended the meaning of the relational third to include how the unconscious subjectivities of both parties cocreate another unconscious structure that is more than the sum of the parts. He called this the *analytic third*. When applied to groups, the analytic third refers to the group's cocreation of the unconscious intersubjective space that is more than the sum of its parts.

With so many thirds, we might say there is a good deal going on! If binary ways of thinking are imposed on group processes—such as contracting for what can and cannot be said or how something must be said—it will give the message that certain forms of subjectivity are desirable or even more normal than others, and the psychological space will be compromised.

The Use of the Third in Group Psychotherapy

My focus here is on my use of the third in the group. In the example described earlier, we left the analyst rather frozen in her thoughts but with one tiny corner of her mind able to think. Using the theory of the third, her thinking represents the metaphorical father or the developmental third, which releases her temporarily from the desire to retaliate. The therapist uses this small mental space to recognise that she needs time to recover from the attack and space to reflect on its meaning, so she asks the group for their reflections on what they see happening. The group represents another developmental third in that their reflections further interpose a space between the therapist and Yvonne, both literally and in the mind of the therapist. The group also represents a cultural third because the subjective experience of group culture is one of working through enactments and following that with reflective process. The relational third has also been invoked as each person's subjective capacity for understanding brings nuanced meaning to the enactment the group members have just witnessed. Through the intersubjective experience of sharing their thoughts and feelings, they create multiple meanings by cocreating many analytic thirds.

In this environment, the therapist is able to find her mind. She notices that among the group members, there is a tendency to be reactive in some of their comments, blaming Yvonne for attacking the therapist. Part of the therapist is pleased about this, but mindful of the potential for splitting and scapegoating, she offers an interpretation to the group, wondering if Yvonne might be acting out a part of everyone's unconscious desire to kill off the therapist (as in a type of group projective identification; Ogden, 1982/1992). The therapist offers her thought not as a definitive interpretation but as another type of third to be reflected on by the group members. This makes the thought less confrontational and allows for reflection rather than any recrimination and guilt they may feel about their aggression toward Yvonne as a way of avoiding their aggression toward the leader.

After an extended period of thought, some group members acknowledge that they do sometimes feel envious of the leader—especially her authority, power, and ability—and would like to destroy her. This leads to some of the group making deeper links with historical experiences of how persons in authority abused their power and of the murderous rage some group members felt as powerless children. As their reflections continued, the group atmosphere changed as fear and aggression mutated into vitality. In a paradoxical way, the group seemed more alive, the atmosphere was lighter, and there was a feeling of camaraderie in the room. It felt as if a monster had escaped from his cell but was not as terrifying as had been imagined. Yvonne looked confused. She had not been punished or scapegoated, and she was uncertain about what this might mean for her. Davies and Frawley (1992) emphasised the importance of "familiarizing the patient with the sadistic introject" and pointed out that the analyst must interpret this sensitively, "without making the patient enormously guilty" (p. 30). Group situations are ideal for supporting this process, but I doubt that we can prevent our patients from feeling guilt, just as we cannot avoid shame and anxiety. For me, there is nothing that cannot be felt and therefore spoken about.

Conclusion

Erskine's article has provided an opportunity for a reflective discussion on relational group processes. While sharing some of his aims for the group and agreeing with his goal of creating the potential for deep connection, not just interpersonal growth, I have offered an alternative perspective on how to achieve these aims. I propose that safety is located not in the interpersonal relatedness but in holding firm boundaries, and that respect is maintained by using the concept of the third as a way of working with the emotional and psychological consequences of confrontations and conflict within the group. By changing the method of working with relational group process, I argue that it makes it more possible for previously unmetabolised experience to be made conscious, thus contributing to the development of a resilient personality.

REFLECTIONS

In this chapter, I explore how boundaries are vital for enabling something dynamic to happen within the therapy session. In this case, it is a group session in which the cocreated third emerges. The inspiration for this article was a session I did with a group during the summer time. There were eight people in the group and the event occurred during a warm summer's evening. I was also inspired by an article written by Richard G. Erskine entitled "Relational Group Process: Developments in a Transactional Analysis Model of Group Psychotherapy." I have always been curious about how Erskine seems to keep a level, calm, and essentially engage in a positive process of psychotherapy. Yet, in this group, something vicious was occurring and I had to muster all the self-control I could manage not to get into the fight with my client. This was all the more likely because her cultural experience was extremely primitive and although not entirely foreign to my cultural experience, there were some significant underlying differences.

Kaufman (1989), in Schore (1994), argued that the therapist must mirror development by actively engaging the identical processes that shape the self. I knew I needed to foster a different developmental direction, but I first needed to allow my experience of her before I could reclaim my mind from the tug toward war which in those moments felt very compelling. As stated in the article, the idea of "the third" in the form of a mentalising process (Fonagy, 2004) enabled me to formulate a question to the group which eased the tension in the air. I think it was a type of affect regulation because the client was confused but calmed by that developmental process; a process she had never had in the tortured and primitive conditions of her childhood in South America.

Chapter 10

When Parting Is Not Such Sweet Sorrow

Helena Hargaden

Hargaden, H. (2010) When Parting Is Not Such Sweet Sorrow. In Life Scripts in Erskine, *R., (ed.) Analysis of Unconscious Relational Patterns. London: Karnac Books.*

Eric Berne's ability to put psychological phenomena into layman's language is particularly evident in his choice of the term "Script" (1961). Script suggests a story line, a plot, dialogue, denouements, comedy or tragedy, stereotype, archetype, and mythology: the very "stuff" of life. Script is simultaneously simple and complex. Script is the implementation of unconscious experiences which have influenced thoughts and feelings about self and other expressed in the form of narrative. Berne originally defined Script as "an unconscious life plan" (Berne, 1966, p. 228). It is tempting to convert the word "plan" into a concrete reality. A combination of affective inquiry into conscious memory, behavioural observation, and cognitive deduction makes it seem as though it is possible to capture Life Script through a linear narrative. Yet even consciousness "is fragmentary, discontinuous, and much too complex and inaccessible to be captured in a singular, true report" (Mitchell, 1993, p. 53). In this chapter, I propose that the main purpose of Script analysis is to elicit the multiple meanings inherent in a person's Life Script. To do this, the psychotherapist has to find an affective link to the client's unconscious. The following case study demonstrates how the nuances and subtle aspects of script dynamics emerge through transferential relatedness between therapist and client. A relational understanding of projective identification provides an affective connection to the relational unconscious leading to deep emotional intimacy between therapist and client in which both participants are changed.

***

When Duncan first came to see me, he said he wanted "some transactional analysis" because he had issues with his wife. He did not need long-term therapy, he said, as he had just completed five years of psychoanalysis and did not want to get into such a commitment again. He reasoned with me that he did not *need* to come to weekly psychotherapy; he wanted, instead, an ad hoc arrangement as he was often away on business. He had the manner of

DOI: 10.4324/9781032266237-11

someone who knew what he was talking about. Although I would normally question such an arrangement I broke my own rules and went along with it. You might well wonder why I was not more skeptical. Why it was that I did not smell a rat? Instead, I was a willing recruit into Duncan's internal world, ready to embark upon a journey where he needed to be in control. I reasoned that he may well know what he was talking about; after all, he had done a serious bout of psychoanalysis. And in some ways he did, because Duncan, without being conscious of it, required an attuned receptivity to his unconscious mental states.

***

I believe that from the beginning of this psychotherapy, there was an unconscious relational connection between therapist and client. This relational connection, although deeply unconscious, was reflected in my willingness to be recruited to his wishes. Unwittingly I showed the type of flexibility that (Bateman & Tyrer, 2004) say is essential when working with someone who has a personality disorder. However this was not my conscious intention when I agreed to Duncan's terms for therapy. Transactional Analysis can be readily applied to short-term contracts so I reasoned that Duncan was quite justified in making a request for a short-term ad hoc contract even though, as an integrative psychotherapist, as well as a transactional analyst, I had mostly worked in the longer term. Instead of insisting that Duncan conform to my way of working, I persuaded myself that it would be interesting to do short-term therapy and to focus on a more cognitive behavioural type of psychotherapy. This was how I convinced myself to proceed with the therapy contract offered or we might say instructed, for that was how it felt, by Duncan.

***

However, it was not to be. When Duncan attempted suicide a few months into the therapy my increasing concerns about the seriousness of his mental condition were validated. We had arrived at a crossroads 12 weeks into therapy. We needed to get off the road and into the woods. We needed to engage with his unconscious. I remonstrated with myself for entering such an uncontained therapeutic contract. I chided myself about what an idiot I had been to accept such a loose and suspicious contract for psychotherapy. But I had been in a "catch twenty two" situation. I had needed to be "an idiot" for the therapy to get underway. From the beginning, Duncan was insistent that he did not want to enter another long-term relationship because he had spent the past five years on the couch (or as it subsequently turned out refusing to go on the couch for most of the time). He needed to be in control, he told me, and I obliged, finding myself quite taken over and controlled. I intuitively felt I needed to go along with his view of things and he has since acknowledged that if I had insisted upon a tighter contract from the beginning, he would have walked. It is as simple as that.

***

Scripts "belong in the realm of transference phenomena, that is, they are derivatives, or more precisely, adaptations, of infantile reactions and experiences .... It is an attempt to repeat in derivative form a whole transference drama, often subdivided in acts" (Berne, 1961, p. 116). It will become clear how the initial stages of this psychotherapy reflected Duncan's earliest, traumatic experiences in infancy. Part of the art of psychotherapy involves the therapist's willingness to take part in the whole transference drama. And of course this will, by its very nature, be unconscious. The unconscious process can only be known "indirectly – and with peculiar effects" (Meier, 1995). My reflections on my early enactment in this psychotherapy find a resource in (Hoffman, 1998) who maintains that we need to feel free to break our own rules, that a spontaneous response is often a creative one, linked to the uniqueness of the therapy. Nevertheless these creative and intuitive acts usually occur within the therapeutic container, after some time has elapsed in which therapist and client can get a sense of each other. Why was I so readily recruited? I think part of the answer to this puzzle lies in the psychological readiness Duncan had already gained in his former psychoanalysis and my respect for that. I had a sense that Duncan had gone as far as he could with his former psychoanalyst and that intuitively he was looking for someone who would be able to go to those places inside of himself that he needed to visit but had never been able to go to before. Williams (2007) observes that the deepest disturbance will be enacted through boundary violations. In those first few months, we had, in effect, unwittingly enacted out the script protocol "the original experiences that pattern an individual's life" (Berne, 1966, p. 302). In Duncan's case, it was the original experiences contained in the unremembered trauma of his earliest experiences.

***

Duncan's earliest experiences: Duncan had been the first born of a young mother, herself emotionally damaged. His father worked as an ambassador to an Eastern European country where brutal revolution had thrown the country into chaos: a bloody and terrifying event, which coincided with Duncan's birth. The circumstances of his birth and his earliest experiences were traumatic; his mother had been paralysed with fear and feelings of inadequacy whilst his father was caught up in an embassy under siege. Women and children are collateral damage. His life would certainly have been under threat as would have been his mother's. Duncan and I had unwittingly cocreated an uncontained and dangerous environment. We had both nearly been killed off: him physically; me emotionally. We had gone through an experience together which had been risky, ill thought through and yet, nonnegotiable, thus, unwittingly, replicating the conditions surrounding his birth: a bloody revolution. Nevertheless because I had been able to accept Duncan for therapy on his own terms, he sensed that I might therefore be responsive to him in ways which would enable him to let me close to him and learn to trust me.

***

After Duncan's attempted suicide, I felt as though someone had put a gun to my head. I was like a blind woman who has suddenly regained her sight. It was now starkly obvious that the lack of therapeutic containment was not the appropriate therapeutic environment for someone with an harmatic (tragic) script. I was now able to say to him unequivocally, that I was unable to work with him unless he came to see me twice a week and in addition joined the therapy group I ran once a week. After such a shock I thought it important I stress my terms. Duncan, subdued, and medicated, acquiesced although I suspected that a part of him would feel deeply resentful about adapting to my way of working. I felt as though I had passed a test. How many more times would I be challenged? The answer was: many.

***

My work with Duncan (alongside collaborative work with other colleagues) influenced my theoretical direction toward the development of relational transactional analysis. In particular the significance of the relational unconscious was clearly, from the beginning, an active part of my relatedness with Duncan. Our connectedness was linked to unconscious aspects of his experience (and, as it subsequently turned out, mine) and can best be understood through the theory of projective identification. In our relational perspective of projective identification (Hargaden & Sills, 2002), we draw upon Ogden's description of projective identification in which he proposes that the infant induces a feeling state in the other that corresponds to a state that he is unable to experience for himself. The recipient allows for the induced state to reside within, and by reinternalising this externally metabolised experience the infant gains a change in the quality of his experience (Ogden, 1992). We refer to this as the "transformational transference." From a relational perspective, the therapist's job involves her linking into what is unconscious in her own mind, a process which involves her in undergoing a change. The impact of the therapist's change impacts upon the mutuality between client and therapist so that the space between them is altered. It is thus a bidirectional process in which the client experiences the therapist in a new and different way, one in which previous experience is contained. In this way, the client and therapist alter each other and formerly unsymbolised experience becomes conscious and tolerable through an interpersonal relationship in which the therapist is willing to change.

***

The theory of projective identification provides a framework for thinking about experiences which, by their very nature, require us to think the unthinkable whilst a relational perspective endorses the role of mutuality in this transferential process. But theory can never prepare us for those times when we are caught up in the eye of the storm. When the twister comes, as in the Wizard of Oz, it carries Dorothy away, turns her world upside down and when she lands in Oz, everything is different. It is at such times that we are caught off guard. Duncan and I often got caught up in a whirlwind of emotional exchange but one day the twister came, taking us over the rainbow and beyond. Would we survive? Unlike hurricanes, most people do not survive the eye of the tornado unless they are in a film called the Wizard of Oz!

***

There had of course been a cumulative buildup to the tensions, which emerged before the day in question. For instance, the theme that stalked the therapy from day one was the issue of ending. Duncan's fear of commitment was a mask for his fear of ending, his anxiety about abandonment, his terror of getting hurt again, and this fear strengthened, deepened, and intensified through the course of a therapy that gradually brought us into deep emotional intimacy. The closer we became, the more he struggled with the ending of the session. He told me this many times in a variety of different ways. He and I thought we could understand why it was so hard for him because of his memories of returning to boarding school at the end of holidays. His dread was so intense that he had tried, with all his might, effort, and will, and every fibre of his being, to make the traffic lights stay on red: forever.

***

He was a particularly sensitive child evidenced in comments made by other members of the family and outsiders. An uncle had returned from taking him to boarding school, pale and shaken, feeling very sad about having had to leave Duncan at the school. An outsider to the family had commented to his father: "your son is a very sensitive young boy." He had been particularly vulnerable to any separation, experiencing it as abandonment, and the subsequent macho life of the school where bullying, humiliation, and fighting were daily occurrences only made it worse. Duncan's earliest experiences had left him with an unbearable sensitivity in which all separations were experienced as intolerable rejections and abandonment. In his relational essay

"Mourning and Melancholia," Freud describes how melancholia is more than just loss of the object:

> It proceeds precisely from those experiences that involved the threat of losing the object. For this reason the exciting causes of melancholia have a much wider range than those of mourning .... In melancholia accordingly, countless separate struggles are carried on over the object, in which hate and love contend with each other; the one seeks to detach the libido from the object, the other to maintain this position of the libido against the assault.
>
> (Freud, 1917, p. 250)

***

Duncan's earliest experiences of object loss and the struggles he encountered as an infant reflect the melancholic process exactly. His experiences of abandonment, yearnings, needs, losses, and terror of near extinction eventually wound their way into the therapy sessions and became particularly pronounced in the way the sessions would end. We never seemed to be able to end on time. Although I would say, "We have now finished," or, "We are ending," or, "Time has run out," or, "So we are ending for today," Duncan would often not move for quite a while. When he did move, it seemed as though he had to drag himself out of the chair. I wondered about it, feeling somewhat paralysed myself about how to think or what to do about it. He began to wonder what I would do if he did not go at the end of sessions. Would I ignore him? Leave him to starve? Throw him the odd crust as he sat in my room wasting away, becoming a skeleton. I too would wonder what I would do. I felt nervous; after all he was over six foot and had had some violent episodes in his past, with his wife. I reflected upon his desperation, his desire, his wondering about how sadistic I would be. For instance would I leave him to die? How compassionate would I be, would I feed him? Would I throw him out? Although it sounded melodramatic these questions were very real for Duncan and indeed for me.

***

When we explored what it meant for him to leave me at the end of sessions, he said that as he walked out of the door, he felt that he lost me, lost the warmth, the connection, the meaning, the life. His experience of abandonment was very stark. A cumulative sense of tension attached itself to this theme when one day he told me that when he left me he sometimes felt so desperate that he parked around the corner, sometimes for one and a half hours, sitting paralysed, unable to move. Letting me know how much I meant to him was a risk, which brought us even closer. Shortly after telling me this I had to move a session from a Thursday to a Friday. On Friday, he told me that he had spent the previous day with his head in his hands, not knowing how he would be able to leave on Friday. I said how it sounded to me that he felt he would be crucified; and that I would be the one to condemn him to his destiny. I reflected on the image of Jesus on the Cross, crying out in despair, "My God! My God! Why Hast Thou Forsaken Me?" I was unsure how this image impacted upon him but it helped me get a sense of the sheer awfulness of the experience he was trying to communicate. I felt moved and helpless at the same time. I felt a huge pressure to do: What? I could not think? I acknowledged his profound sense of despair and desperation but such a transaction felt too trite for he already knew how he felt. I elaborated upon the metaphor of the crucifixion to empathise with his experience of isolation and bleakness. I expressed my sadness about such a forlorn state of affairs but none of it made any difference to his desperate sense of abandonment. Neither empathy nor interpretation was sufficient.

***

Some authors write as if the patient's subjective experience can simply be uncovered, allowed to unfold in a receptive, empathic environment, much as Freud thought the analyst's neutrality allowed the patient's intrapsychic conflicts to emerge in an uncontaminated fashion. They overlook the extent to which the patient is always speaking selectively to a particular other person for a specific purpose.

(Mitchell, 1993, p. 69)

***

Here, Mitchell points out the limitations of a one-person psychology whether that is a humanistic one with its emphasis on empathy as the "curative" factor, or psychoanalysis with its emphasis upon detachment and interpretation as the crucial ingredient in cure.

These features of detachment, interpretation, and empathy are of course significant aspects of psychotherapy but we are left with the question: "*How* do we convey our understanding as psychotherapists?"

***

We got closer to the crux of the matter when Duncan said one day, "I just don't know how you can do it! How can you send me away at the end of the session? If you truly understood how I feel you would not do it. Oh, yes, of course I know intellectually why you do it," he said despairingly, "but it makes no difference to me."

***

Words alone were clearly not deepening our communication. Duncan felt unmoved by my words whether they were shaped into metaphors, interpretations, or reflected his feelings. Words became like a strait jacket between us, full of sound and fury, but often not able to signify the meaning. Many words were uttered, creating noise and sound but thudding onto the floor, at the end of sessions, leaving a sense that all we had said was as nothing as compared to an unnamable "something." In some ways, the volume of words captured the impossibility of communication between us. I sensed, with some dread, that we were gradually and inexorably moving toward an impasse. This is how impasses occur, slowly, subtly: with difficulty and a degree of certainty we moved toward our dichotomous positions.

***

Moments of meeting: Moments of change are sometimes referred to as "aha moments." Daniel Stern describes them as "moments of meeting" in which "each partner has actively contributed something unique and authentic of his or herself as an individual (not unique to their theory or technique of therapeutics) in the construction of the "moment of meeting" (Stern, 1998, p. 913). To the untrained ear, these moments can seem unremarkable. One has to listen to the recounting of these moments with a certain sensibility. We need to be attuned to the bi directionality of the relational unconscious; how we shape each other at every turn; that unless the therapist allows this shaping she cannot change. If she cannot change, then no change will be possible. Yet not only must she be shaped and changed, but also she has to find a way of thinking about what is happening and how to choose the words that will matter. We cannot plan for moments of meeting when the intensity of exchange is at its height; we need to improvise. At the mercy of our integrity, pushed to the limits of our creative capacity, we realise we have come to the end of our theory and have dived into the sea of feelings (Eigen, 2007). Such moments invariably involve us in the dilemma about self-disclosure. Even as we unconsciously reveal ourselves, we still have choices about what to verbally disclose.

How to convey those moments of meeting? Duncan shuddered as he came into the room; I cannot go there again he said portentously. I must not make him leave, he said emphatically. I asked him why he thought I "made" him leave and he said, quick as a flash, that it was my inhuman part which made him go. That if I understood the pain he was in, how excruciating it was, how his head hurt and as he spoke he again had a vivid recollection of willing the traffic lights to stay on red as he was being driven back to the boarding school, screaming inside with pain—but, he wailed, they never did, even now, seeming to be anguished by his inability to stop the dreaded journey. "So, why do you make me go?" He said insistently. He was clearly not in the mood for me to stay in a mode of enquiry into his mental states, to hear metaphors, interpretations, or receive empathy. Instead, I was to be put on the spot. I felt anxious. What on earth would I do if he did not move? What about the next client? How would I get him out of his chair? Under threat and unable to think, I grabbed a thought out of the air which conveniently presented itself to me as a plausible one: "It is an existential issue" I said, importantly and firmly, hoping this would provide containment. He looked at me with contempt—quite rightly so as it was a pathetic response, I now readily concede. If not exactly an inhuman one, he experienced it thus, and indeed it was at least a rather detached offering. In hock to my severe sense of anxiety, I had attempted to set a boundary by pulling rank and citing a technical term, which I hoped would subdue him. The tension in the air was palpable. His long legs were stretched out ahead of him, nearly touching me, as I sat still in my chair, feeling completely stuck. I had no idea what to say, my mind went blank: I could barely think. I started to feel sick, and overcome with tiredness. I thought I might throw up and started wondering about what I had had for breakfast. That thought jolted me into Adult awareness. This was somatic countertransference, I reasoned, but it made no difference to my nausea. I had to escape. I had enough presence of mind to translate my experience into a half appropriate intervention: "I need to put a pause button on the session," I said. I have a tickle in my throat, and need to leave the room to get some water. The colour of his eyes deepened with scorn, and as I followed the trajectory of his eyes moving from me to a space beside my chair my heart beat faster as I heard him say, there's a bottle of water by your chair. Oh, said I, with false brightness, so there is and I picked it up and took a long swig, the way a condemned prisoner might ask for one last drink before being lead away to the gallows: to my untimely fate.

***

But the action was enough to change the atmosphere in the room. We had moved out of a direct relationship into one in which we talked *about* our relationship. I felt much better, the sickness went and I was curious to see where he was in himself. The tension had subsided. "So what do you think was going on between us just then?" I asked. He said, "Well I think you used the water as a diversionary tactic to get us out of the mess we were in and it has worked because I am no longer feeling the pain of being inside that place."

What a sensitive man he is, I thought! He knows I have "bottled" it and he is annoyed. I tried to get back to the former situation. "Let us revisit that experience then," I said. But, he said, he couldn't, so I said, "well let's talk about it." He knew I had made a mistake and I felt that he was punishing me for it but now, more restored by the water and the reduction in tension, I persisted. "How do you understand what was going on between us?" He answered, "Well you were damned no matter what I said, because you could not get past the question: how can you send me away if you really understand my painful feelings?" As he said this, once more his face contorted as he reconnected with his pain.

***

I was reconnected with my ability to think and be in the present moment: reconnected with my Adult ego state: back in my mind. I felt also a sense of being back in my body; my sickness had gone. From this experience of embodiment, I was able to recognise that I needed separation and space to take my time to engage with Duncan's question; something I could not do when I felt hounded by his urgent and enraged requests for answers. I need time to think about it, I said. I need time to reflect. We sat together in silence, and I began to reflect upon his question. As I did so I began to feel tearful. A random memory came to me of when my younger son clung on to my coat to try and stop me leaving him at nursery. I had felt heartbroken at the time. I remembered it well. I thought about loss, the pain of it. A recent article came into my mind, by Darien Leader, a psychoanalyst, and author of a book entitled *The New Black* (Guardian, 2008). Leader makes a scathing attack upon the cultural obsession with "depression" and the use of drugs to treat what really would be more accurately understood as the effects of mourning or melancholia. Leader refers to Freud's 1917 essay on Mourning and Melancholia. Leader had reminded me of Freud's essay and I had recently reread it several times. As I sat here with Duncan, I reflected on what I had read.

***

Freud describes the difference between mourning and melancholia in which both have the same symptoms. He says the main difference is that melancholia is unconscious: "that melancholia is in some way related to an object-loss which is withdrawn from consciousness, in contradistinction to mourning, in which there is nothing about the loss that is unconscious" (Freud, 1917. p. 254). Mourning is therefore a conscious process whereas melancholia is linked to developmental losses about which we often know nothing consciously. Melancholia is the basis of narcissism. Instead of mourning, the person introjects the lost object and turns it against himself the result of which the person is left feeling low self-esteem, and with a deeply destructive hatred of self. He describes the distinguishing mental features of melancholia as

> a profoundly painful dejection, cessation of interest in the outside world, loss of the capacity to love, inhibition of all activity, and a lowering of the self-regarding feelings to a degree that find utterance in self-reproaches and self-revilings, and culminates in a delusional expectation of punishment.
>
> (Freud, 1917, p. 252)

Freud's essay is very helpful to the psychotherapist in making such a distinction because it enables an empathic response to the melancholic state of narcissism.

Freud's essay points us in the direction of looking for *what* was lost and helps shape our countertransference when we may be inclined to feel callous, indifferent, irritated and impatient. So, LOSS is at the bottom of it all. Loss of so many things, both unknown, known and ongoing. A simple sounding word yet so painful when we really engage with our losses. Freud said that life is difficult and that loss will always be painful; there is no way of making loss not painful. Bob Dylan (1967) describes Love as a four-letter word but at that moment I thought it is Loss, which is also a four-letter word. *Loss is always painful. Loss is always painful.* Those words were like a refrain.

***

As I sat with Duncan deep in thought I felt the sorrow of life's losses, feeling both soothed and moved by the wisdom and simplicity of Freud's words.

***

I was then able to know what I really wanted to say to Duncan. I told him that how, when we parted, I felt the loss of him. "It is not just the loss of you," I said, "but when I feel the loss of you at the end of our sessions, it gets into all of my other losses, and it hurts; sometimes I cut it off, because I too don't want to feel the pain of it." As I said these words, it occurred to me, for the first time, how traumatised I sometimes felt at the end of sessions with Duncan, where, at those times when there was space, I would sit in front of my laptop aimlessly playing a card game, in a paralysed condition, sometimes for up to half an hour. Duncan looked at me with astonishment. "My God, why do you do this job?" I felt vulnerable and exposed and thought to myself with feeling: "why *do* I do this job?" In the spirit of the depth of honest exchange that had emerged, I said, "Because I love it, and because I have had many losses, and in engaging with the pain of those losses, I continue to feel healed by working with people who have also suffered losses which feel intolerable and unbearable." He gave a joyful laugh. His face had changed, his body looked different, and he seemed full of life. "I feel that you have hugged me," he said, smiling, and said he wanted to hug me back. "How extraordinary," he said, "you are extraordinary."

***

You might think, oh dear, "idealization" but as Richard Erskine has pointed out (Erskine, Moursund, & Trautmann, 1998), idealisation is the client's unconscious request for protection. Of course Duncan was, at this point in the therapy, idealising me. He needed my 'extraordinary' understanding and protection from the infant's abandonment by his mother's emotional distress during the revolution and the child's abandonment to the boarding school. For Duncan, it was a truly extraordinary thought and experience, that it was possible to feel one's losses, feel the pain of them, and the vulnerability of it, and, at the same time to not be ashamed of feeling so painfully vulnerable. He had also discovered something quite extraordinary about me: I had a heart! I was like the tin man in the Wizard of Oz, who finds he has a heart after the tornado had taken Dorothy and her companions to a new place. We too had both moved into a new place where I had become a human being. And if I was extraordinary, then, so was he, although we may ask why, after all, is it so extraordinary to mourn our losses? According to Leader (2008), it has indeed become an extraordinary thing to acknowledge and feel the vicissitudes of living instead of reaching for something, anything, which promises to take away our pain. He believes that this has become increasingly pandered to by a culture that seems not to want to recognise the place of mourning in life and that life is hard.

***

Further Reflections: Since Freud (1917), subsequent research into infant development (Stern, 1986, 1998) and the development of neuroscience and the links made to development of the brain (Schore, 1994) have supported Freud's idea of unconscious loss as the root of melancholia. Freud referred to this as losses which are unconscious but affect us in the here and now. When Duncan's losses were not readily available through memory, he found a convincing script narrative in his remembered experiences of boarding school. Erskine (2008) has also shown in his examples how our earliest experiences contribute to representations of interpersonal (object) relationships but do not form a part of a remembered narrative. However these memories alone could not account for the intensity of Duncan's sense of abandonment, a feature which was also commented upon by the family friend, who recognised a traumatised soul and described it as a type of sensitivity. The boarding school experience provided Duncan with a narrative in the absence of conscious declarative memory. It is therefore essential that any serious script analysis take into consideration countertransferential phenomenon as a route through to the client's nonverbalised experience. In the case of Duncan, the only way to gain access to his earliest object relations was through the intensity of the exchange between us. His earliest wishes and fantasies reveal themselves through his wondering aloud with me how I would treat him if he refused to go. "Would I leave him to die? Would I save him? Would I love him? Would I hate him?" I struggled to be open enough to engage with Duncan at this level. I worried for my safety, for example, what would I do if he refused to leave, initially ignoring Duncan's attempts to relive unrepeatable Script experiences. But Duncan was intelligent and he trusted in his intuitions and the promptings from his unconscious. He needed to access my unconscious mental functioning and when I allowed it to happen, when I could eventually share my mind with him and admit my vulnerability and humanness, it brought about a deep emotional intimacy between us. This experience changed him and me. We both knew each other differently after this exchange and nothing could turn the clock back. When I referred back to this session several meetings later,

Duncan had only a dim memory of what had happened. He said that it was misty, reminding me of Monet's impressionistic, misty, but impactful paintings. It was unusual for Duncan not to remember details but as he said the word "misty," his eyes filled, his face softened, and his body relaxed as though he was reliving the experience of connectedness once more.

***

Impasses are an essential and predictable part of any psychotherapy. They will naturally occur as the tension between the past and the present merge through the therapeutic relationship. Yet, when caught in the vortex of the tornado it can be very difficult to think. We need a degree of freedom and we need to learn how to think in those moments. I got stuck in the tension between us; the inhumanness that Duncan had experienced in his infancy and at the boarding school was mirrored in the transferential relationship. The projective identification initially evoked a traumatised part of my psyche in which I could not receive Duncan's loss. All I could manage was the emotionally removed response that felt callous and inhuman in much the same manner that Duncan had once experienced his misattuned mother and his absent father. He tries to reach another part in me but all he gets is the icy and unresponsive part: "It is a question," I say, "of the existential." How icy can you get?! I am sickened maybe by my inability to be humane, I don't wish to know about my icy, callous part. Maybe my disturbance and sickness is about the experience of the bad object in me, the part which mirrors him and is so accurately observed by Duncan when he notes how I used a "diversionary tactic" to get away from him. Duncan brought to my attention previously disassociated parts of my suffering and melancholic preoccupation.

***

It is only when I get back my mind, and connect with my reflective capacity, that I find my humanity and am able to communicate with Duncan in a way he can receive. For Duncan, no platitudes would do, no "therapeutic" interpretations, no fabricated compassion would reach him: he needed truth—he needed to make me into a human being, into someone who could reflect. He not only made me reach my humanity but also made me recognise my inhumanity too: a part which sickens me and makes me want to escape from myself. "It takes one to know one." Duncan and I share similar traits. He has made me recognise that nothing really changes unless the therapist changes. I had to yield and let myself be known in a non defended way.

***

In this Script analysis, projective identification enabled Duncan and I to communicate at a very deep level of emotional intimacy. From a relational perspective, I worked with the projective identification by engaging with my self-states which are, as we have seen, unique to my Script. Someone else sitting with Duncan would have done something quite different. For instance they may have been more inclined to stay with Duncan's experience of the therapist's inhumanity and explore his experience from that perspective. The point was that I had stopped thinking, because he had engaged my inhuman part so successfully. His experience of my vulnerability, his access to my unconscious enabled Duncan to change his Script and to feel, at last, understood and to let go of the shame which had haunted him all his life for feeling so weakened by his vulnerability. For the first time, Duncan was able to leave, feeling that he carried me with him, instead of losing me at the door.

REFLECTIONS

The inspiration for this chapter came from the unusual circumstances of how the therapy began, which is described in the article. There were so many twists and turns in the story that it made for a compelling case study. I came to recognise the depth of agony he had experienced as an infant and, thereafter, from his narrative. Over the course of 20 years, I helped to grow him and he became a very dear and beloved client. Because we understand so much about the interpersonal world of the infant who is seeking attunement and mirroring, I recognised from the story of his birth, born into a raging European war, that Charles' experience of the world was one of coldness, terror, and a threat of extinction. Shakespeare captures the root of the paradox that operated continuously in our work. With me, he was finding happiness in his experience of validation, companioning, reasoning, affective regulating; but, when we parted, he lost me. Only when he could find me within himself could he rest easy.

Chapter 11

To Be or Not to Be—Is That the Question? The Paradox of Script

Helena Hargaden

I am honoured to be opening this conference. "To be or not to be" is perhaps the most iconic phrase in the English language. It not only is a part of our cultural heritage but also captures the universal existential dilemma of existence. For this reason, I think that to be or not to be *is* the question; and what I have to say today links this phrase to be or not to be with the paradox embodied in script, the challenges involved in vulnerability, and the creative opportunities available from engaging with diversity of theoretical perspectives.

As psychologists, we are of course tuned in to the existential dilemma of to be or not to be. Indeed within transactional analysis, there are specific models of theory, which enable us to focus on precisely the dilemma of existence. Of course, this dilemma poses more questions for us than just survival, what do we do and how do we do it once we do make the decision "to be," becomes increasingly more complex. Shakespeare asks this very question, "Whether 'tis nobler in the mind to suffer the slings and arrows of outrageous fortune, Or to take arms against a sea of troubles, And by opposing end them?" The paradox of life is that we choose "to be" in the knowledge that one day will shuffle "off this mortal coil." How to live knowing we will die is a part of the existential dilemma I would suggest that underlies all script decisions.

In thinking about the paradox of script, we can find much to teach us in most of Shakespeare's plays but in particular, Hamlet. When Shakespeare wrote this play, he had just lost his father, and his infant child, Hamnet had also just died. He was in grief. In his book *The New Black,* Darien Leader says to grieve means we need to do something, to be creative. Well Shakespeare certainly did that with his play Hamlet; it could even be seen as a prayer, a hymn, an incantation, a poem, an outpouring of his grief as he wrestled with "the slings and arrows of outrageous fortune" himself.

Some years ago I was interested to come across a book entitled, *Shakespeare, The invention of the Human,* by Harold Bloom, which I found very informative from a psychological perspective. In his chapter on Hamlet, Bloom describes the play as a celebration of the inner world. The play is full

DOI: 10.4324/9781032266237-12

of pain, loss, suffering, ghosts, murderous rage, anger sadness, loss, destruction.betrayals, very similar indeed to the type of treacherous psychological journey many of us have undergone, and which we invite our clients to partake in, when we offer them the opportunity to go on a journey of relational depth. Bloom says,

> Hamlet as a character, bewilders us because he is so endlessly suggestive. Are there any limits to him? His inwardness is his most radical originality, the ever-growing inner self, the dream of an infinite consciousness, has never been more fully portrayed.

This comment by Bloom made me think about Hamlet as a type of prototype of the psychotherapist, was he the first psychotherapist looking to develop his consciousness to its limits? Bloom describes Hamlet as the Western hero of consciousness. He says that "the internalisation of the self is one of Shakespeare's greatest inventions." For me Hamlet's mystery, his real interiority, preempts the relational psychotherapist, who seeks to know her own interiority, to acknowledge the mystery of this work, and to become as self aware as is possible to be. In Hamlet, we see a man whose whole world is the growing inner self, which he sometimes attempts to reject, but which nevertheless he celebrates.

In thinking about Bloom's stimulating and scholarly work on Shakespeare's scripts, I am reminded again how the TA idea of Script is pure genius. It makes intuitive and cognitive sense to think about peoples' lives in the context of having a script. Of course, there are many ways to look at a script. Hamlet is testimony to this. There are many different interpretations of Hamlet and his soliloquies. What did he mean? What was he trying to say? How do we understand him? These are questions that have never been fully answered because they cannot be. There is no linear way to understand Hamlet; no linear way to understand humanness.

When I was asked to do this keynote speech my mind wandered to my past. I recalled how the play Hamlet was a massive force for positivity in my life. The circumstances which led to this were linked to a powerful script decision I made on a summer's evening when I was 16; a script decision that was truly paradoxical in terms of its potential for goodness and negativity in my life as you will see from the following story.

When I was ten years old, my immigrant parents sent me to a private Roman Catholic Convent School. Like many immigrants, they wanted their children to be better than them, to be educated. But also like many immigrants, they were a bit chaotic in their thinking and went on to have two more babies making us a family of six—four children and two adults. This meant that they found it difficult to pay the fees and struggled with having a larger family. I was at the school for five years and for most of that time I rebelled. It must have been a fairly intelligent rebellion because I kept just enough below the radar to prevent being expelled although some of my closest friends were expelled. It was a very strict school. My rebellions took the form of taking my much hated hat off as soon as I got outside the school gates, wearing the badge at the back instead of the front of the hated hat, sitting through a physics exam in the science lab, and instead of trying to answer the questions, drawing a rabbit which was sitting outside of the window (my drawing abilities were zilch); very often sitting at the back of the class, not doing my homework, refusing to catch the hard hurting rounders' ball when the PE teacher (much disliked by me) screamed, catch that ball girl! while I silently had no intention of hurting myself by catching, what I thought of, as her ball.

Of course, these petty rebellions were all distractions from my unhappy state of mind. Consciously unhappy because of the unpaid fees, required to look after babies when I was trying to grow into a young woman, the loss of security linking me unconsciously to my infant experiences of hospitalisation and the abandonment and loss involved, which of course I only understood after being in therapy. After five years, the Head Nun had had enough of me and told my mother at the schools gates, I recall it well, the lovely old buildings in the background, us at the end of the elegant driveway, her clasping my mother's hand, saying, "I think it best that Helena does a bit of typing before she gets married and has children." Well, she could hardly have said a better thing to a very rebellious girl. In many ways, the life I have led has been spurred on by her lack of aspiration for me and my script decision to rebel against it. And, I have three degrees, and many diplomas to prove it! I made a powerful script decision to go against the message to not succeed. A very significant part of that script decision was my parents' attitude to this patronising and insulting directive by the Head Nun. They were very angry and called the head nun names I cannot repeat here. This only helped buffer my decision to prove her wrong. My Child Ego state was further supported by their rebellions Child, so the Parent in my Child, combined with my own child took up a position against the super ego, the Parent ego state embodied by the nun. The fact that my script decision was supported by my parents resulted in a much better prognosis for me than if they had sided with her. I will come back to say a bit more about this script decision later.

But first to say a bit more about what happened to me after leaving school with no qualifications and how it came that I found Hamlet. I went to a secretarial college, and duly did typing, shorthand, English O levels in language and literature, business studies and excelled (rebelliously) in them all; then went to London where I worked as a temporary secretary, which meant I could change jobs on a whim, and earn a high hourly fee. During the day I was what was then described as a dolly bird, with false eyelashes and mini skirt (all part of my rebellion against my Catholic upbringing). In the evenings, dressed more casually, together with my best friend Pat, we met up with Irish lads from Galway in our local pub in Earls Court called The Prince of Tech where we used to get drunk and talk about the meaning of life. They were drop outs from Galway University and in our drunken conversations, they used to tell me how I was wasted as a secretary and I should go to university. I found their advice, quite encouraging and acceptable since it came from the drop out boys from Galway, a comradely cell of rebellion, chiming as it did with my rebel child.

Some years later, bored stiff, I took the boys' advice and returned to Central College in Liverpool where I was told I could study O levels in a year and then A levels, all in all taking three years. I found this rather discouraging but found out I could do something called the Mature Matriculation, which involved choosing the subjects you wished to study at university and taking an intensive examination in those subjects at the end of the year. I chose English literature and philosophy. I thought philosophy was more akin to psychotherapy (not that I knew that word at the time) so was appalled to be given the book, Language Truth and Logic by A.J. Ayer, based on logical positivism, meaning you cannot know anything unless it is verified. But for the English Literature exam I was given Hamlet to study. In essence, I had two books to study, which were at opposite ends of the mental spectrum: logical positivism in which nothing is real unless it can be verified and the other, opening up the realm of metataphysical enquiry, questioning the very nature of reality, portraying a world where there are are barely any identifiable facts. Determined to succeed, still in rebellious mode, I studied both. I read Hamlet inside out and back to front, bought the Long Playing Vinyl with Sir Gielgud playing Hamlet and read all the literary critiques I could find.

The paradox of my rebelliousness was that it brought me into the world of education but not only that, it was in studying Hamlet that I first learned the ground rules in how to think about psychotherapy and Script. Those of you who have studied English Literature will know that it is based largely on the idea of critiquing script and texts. I found numerous and very different critiques of Hamlet. Peopled argued learnedly and even ferociously over the meaning of the play, and of Hamlet's soliloquies. It was here I first learned the ground rules in how to think about psychotherapy and Script. For the major theme in all of Shakespeare's plays is the difference between appearance and reality, the difference between the social and the psychological; the difference between the surface and the depth. When studying Hamlet I learned to ask questions about the nature of his script?

What is reality? What is real? Is he a murderer? Is he destructive? What is the real story here? Maybe there isn't just one story? Maybe there are multiple truths? Maybe life cannot be easily understood in linear ways. After reading 21 different interpretations of Hamlet, I called it a day. I had enough material to do my exam. Fortunately for me AJ Ayer's book brooks only one interpretation. It was in studying Hamlet that I learned to play with the dialectic of different interpretations I had found, to learn that the only truths are paradoxical ones, to think for myself, on the one hand this and on the other hand that to make up my own mind. This is where I first learned to stay and play with the nature of ambiguity—the role of uncertainty is of course central to working with script from a relational perspective.

Here I wish to refer to a philosophical essay entitled "The Ambiguity of Ethics" published in *Les Tempes Moderne*, in 1947, by Simone de Beauvoir. In this essay, De Beauvoir maintains the existentialist belief in absolute freedom of choice and the consequent responsibility that such freedom entails. She argues that when we project power into institutions systems or people we subordinate our freedom (that would of course include governments, institutions of any type, systems, organisations, theories, or people including families.) Rather than embracing our freedom to think for ourselves, she argues, we lose it in what she describes as a type of bad faith. If we extend this understanding to psychological theory, it is easy to see how reifying theory, by giving it power such as classical TA or relational TA or any TA or any psychological theory, or logical positivism, makes it more likely that we lose the motivation or need to take responsibility for ourselves and instead hide our vulnerability behind theoretical concepts. De Beauvoir maintains that in projecting our power into systems and people in this way the system becomes ever more mystical and oppressive, claiming to represent the natural order of things. We know this from within our own profession where for example Freud, or Rogers, Ferenzi, or Berne, is deemed by their apostles to have the final word on truth, and it is in this way that relatedness and relationship are forced into concrete ideas, as if permanent, when we lose the right to be able to critique, have an independent mind, and workout our own standpoints.

Of course when we no longer project outward into systems, theories, or people we are reliant upon power from within. Naturally this makes us more vulnerable if we are not hiding behind something, someone. For the relational therapist, her vulnerability is the source of her power.

Let me tell you a story from my practice, about 25 years ago, which illustrates the power of the therapist's vulnerability. It is taken from my new book, *The Art of Relational Supervision, Clinical Implications of the Use of the Self in Supervision Groups* in which six members of supervision groups I have led over the years have contributed very interesting accounts of their vulnerability as therapists. In the following short vignette from my practice, I recall my work with a man who was possibly on the autistic spectrum, a condition I was unfamiliar with at the time. He spoke through the medium of his fascination and love for the composer Bartok, speaking in detail about Bartok's use of tonality, which apparently did not follow traditional lines of musicality. His detailed description of the numerical aspects of the music often sounded like arithmetic or algebra to my ears. I made a mental note never to listen to this composer. With the benefit of hindsight and experience, I can now see that he was trying to tell me something in code about his difficulty with emotional connecting. Impervious to this understanding at the time I tried to decipher what he was saying through the medium of my fascination with the theoretical perspectives of transactional analysis and person-centred psychotherapy. So my response to my client's communication was to jump up quite frequently to a whiteboard, and draw circles and triangles on the board, referring to ego states (Berne, 1961) and the drama triangle (Karpman, 1968), trying, as I imagined, to respond empathically to what my client was telling me by converting it into circles and triangles and doing quite a bit of talking. We must have looked a rather odd couple; him with his algebra and arithmetic and me with my geometry. To an onlooker, it would have seemed as though we were speaking in "tongues"! Nonetheless something important was happening but I had no consciousness of what that might be then.

About three months into the treatment, on the night before his session, my small son was ill and I spent a sleepless and anxious night tending to him. I cannot recall what the illness was but I was very uneasy and all the more so because any child's illness made me fearful and excessively anxious of pending loss, again with the unconscious echo of my time spent in hospital as an infant, not that I thought about that at the time. Instead of cancelling the session, I stoically carried on. However I was not in my "fascinated with my theory" mode. Instead I was feeling vulnerable, and in the type of space between sleep and wakefulness, that the poet John Keats (1899) described as "negative capability," the mental twilight zone when the poet is at his most creative. In this vulnerable state, I was more reliant on my intuitive sense and although I cannot recall what exactly I said. I was most conscious, however, of a feeling of discomfort that I was not doing my job properly and hoping my client did not notice that I was not talking so much. I was surprised, when, at the end of the session, my client stood up, picked up his brief case and, turning to face me, and, after a pause, when it seemed that he might be deciding whether to comment or not, and in which I dreaded to hear the words that he was leaving therapy, he thanked me for the session, saying, "that was our best session yet." I could see the feeling in his eyes, and something about the vulnerability of his body was captured by the way his pinstriped suit seemed to wrap itself around him, reminding me of how an infant is protected in a shawl, leaving me with feeling a deep sense of sadness as he left.

Feelings had finally got through to me; feelings he had been trying to convey in his obsession with Bartok's unconventional use of tonality. It seemed, that it was the quality of my listening, infused by the uncertainty that sleeplessness can bring, and an attuned sensibility toward the physical and mental sickness in myself and others, which most affected him. I sat with my reflections, I noticed another emotion which was at odds with my sense that I had not done a very good job, it was a sense of my worth and value in those moments of meeting between us: my value as a human being. Something had happened that I had no theory for then; something which was intriguing and encouraging, leading me to think that maybe it was possible to be a good clinician while I strayed outside the strait jacket of theoretical constructions.

Of course, this demand to consider myself of value took time. Going back to by script decision. The rebellious child eventually hit a brick wall behind which was a crumbling edifice, beyond which I could go no further and many years in Jungian analysis brought me to my knees, struggling through the debris, rubble, and lack of foundation hidden under the rebellion, to search for what was really valuable, learning how to be, just to be, of value.

How do we listen to narratives? How to find the true meaning of scripts. In the aforementioned story, my vulnerability seeped out against my will, and fortunately the client was so boundaried and difficult to penetrate, he was able to use it to his psychological advantage. For of course the work of using, the therapist's vulnerability in the service of the client is a very complex process involving a depth of nuanced attunmenet, discernment and breath of knowledge to manage and contain such moments of meeting therapeutically. But this experience was the first step in beginning to use my soul and heart, and not just work from the theory driven head.

To be or not to be, for me is the question, it is the great existential question that we can either relate to and engage with or disavow; either way has consequences for how we live our lives of course.

In this keynote speech, I have spoken from my heart and my head, combined. You will have noticed that throughout the speech, I have referred to the relational perspective: this is because I have spent much of my time as a psychotherapist, developing this approach to my work. From this perspective I do not think there is a question of to be classical or not to be classical, to be relational or not to be relational. To be both, or to be neither? By the relational approach, I mean to describe more a sensibility than a set of theories. For me, the relational approach involves a living process between theory and ourselves, that is *what* we do and *how* we do it, but it should never involve us forcing relatedness into idee fixee. It involves a continuous search to find new language that paves the way for more nuanced and in depth ways to examine our subjective experiences. It involves us in the rights to our existential choices, and acts of freedom in the therapy encounter. Today, I have emphasised the truth embodied in paradox, the power of vulnerability, and the mystery inherent in our work. No one tribe or creed has a monopoly on good ideas. The best work is the fusion of all of us.

For me difference involves a dialectical relationship between multiple perspectives.

Let us all, in this creative and vital TA community, keep a dialogue between different ways of thinking, working, being together, open to play with the dialectic, keep ourselves open to critiquing, to thinking, to working out our own standpoints, and not to give our power away to any one person, theory, or organisation. Let us have a good conference.

REFLECTIONS

In the case study described I had previously, done one year of training in person-centred counselling. When I think back to this occasion, I am vividly reconnected with my body as though I am once more in the room with this man. It is now 30 years since I saw him; yet, I just know him in my heart, mind, and body. As I recount, in this talk, I was awake all night with a sick child. What I failed to grasp, because I had not done my in-depth psychotherapy, was that I was transported back to two hospital experiences I had as a new born and then one-year old. After trying to understand the client by using circles, and him using Bartok the composer, we united in a type of empathic immersion as I listened to him from a completely different set of "self states." He felt it; and it was during those moments and in the aftermath, when he told me it was the best session to date, that, I now realise, the genesis of my relational understanding took root.

So now I can think about what happened in that room so many years ago. We were both communicating from our right brain–right brain connection. There is no doubt. But, at the time, without this knowledge, I was unable initially to recognise what was happening between us. After this occasion, I "pulled myself together," reverted to circles, and he continued with Bartok, only to leave a short time later as we were unable to reconnect at this level. I had received information that I could not value at the time. I had operated from deeply felt knowledge in my right hemisphere that was not yet conscious to me, so I could do nothing with it. "Feelings are poised at the very threshold that separates being from knowing and thus have a privileged connection to consciousness" (Damasio, 1999, p. 49). The client tried to teach me something and I tried to listen, but I was very far from valuing my knowledge or making meaning out of it and reverted to my left hemispheres "knowledge" without the assistance of my right hemisphere. The left hemisphere with its circles and facts, therefore, became redundant after a while. It just was not enough.

In my talk, I quote from Hamlet who, according to Bloom (1999), was the prototype of the first therapist, in his struggles, depth of uncertainty, straining toward the "truth," looking to find meaning. In this way, Hamlet shows us the type of journey we embark upon if we wish to do depth psychotherapy. And of course most of us do! For what use is cognitive behavioural change when what can be altered this way easily can revert back again after six months or so? Shakespeare was the first dramatist to offer us a multidimensional view of the human being. He puts his characters on stage and reveals to us their internal worlds though the use of soliloquy in which we begin to recognze the inside from the outside, as we see the character behaving so differently when with another person.

Iago, (THE CORRECT NAME IS IAGO) for example, reveals his true self from his persona, which is seductive and meant to convince Othello of Desdemona's betrayal. The therapist has to find a way of being true to herself in all her different aspects if she is to be any use as a psychotherapist.

> *This above all: to thine own self be true,*
> *And it must follow, as the night the day,*
> *Thou canst not then be false to any man.*
> William Shakespeare
> "Hamlet" Act 1, Scene 3, 78–82

Chapter 12

A Talk on Money, Race, and the links with Karpman's Triangle

Helena Hargaden

Given for the 2009 Relational Psychoanalytic Conference, London.

Next I share some rumination, a brief case study, and finally some questions with which to play.

Money is currently a very hot issue (some might say when is it not!) because of the last few years of crisis in the money markets. On a radio programme recently, someone rang in to ask the question: Where does money come from? The answer was: the central banks of the world who print the money, which raises a whole pile of questions for economists, but, the presenter added, that there was a large psychological component in how money worked.

We, in this profession, are not strangers to that idea. At the very least, we can understand money as energy, and as a transactional process in which something is exchanged for money. Money inevitably raises issues about worth and value and valuing. Money is, therefore, both concrete and symbolic. This is not groundbreaking news for psychotherapists; but, money raises specific areas of exploration for us.

We are required to reflect on cultural views about money; explore as far as possible unconscious attitudes both from the collective unconscious and our own hidden Script issues. In the collective unconscious, there are archetypal influences upon us of which we strive to become conscious. For instance, my very first thoughts when I was asked to be on this panel to discuss money were biblical sayings about money, such as "money is the root of all evil" and that famous one about "the camel, the rich man, and the eye of a needle"! It is relatively easy to come to the primitive conclusion that rich = bad, and poor = good.

These archetypes hover on the periphery of our awareness, as do our own Script decisions and experiences of money. For instance, how our parents talked about money and how, as a family, we dealt with money. In my experience, many families have a culture of deficit and scarcity in their stories; no matter how rich, it can feel that catastrophe is just around the corner. My richest relative reproved the children when growing up for putting too much parmesan on their pasta—did they not know it was very expensive?!

DOI: 10.4324/9781032266237-13

Psychotherapists, of course, spend a considerable amount of time bringing unconscious issues to the foreground. Our own issues of worth and value usually surface in any in-depth analysis of our Script and we expect of ourselves to be conscious that we have an unconscious which cannot be controlled—that unfriendly aspects of self lurk in our shadows. Perhaps one of our most difficult shadows, as a helping profession, is that we prefer to see ourselves as healers, people who are concerned with troubled minds and wish to bring about transformation. This can feel incompatible with the requirements to run a business, to be an entrepreneur, fix fees, do accounts, set boundaries of time and place, and so on. We do not wish to be in anyway seen as horrid, greedy, for example, or uncaring about someone's difficult financial situation. But one thing we know is that money will get into our deepest script issues and our clients, and so these seminars are useful to raise our consciousness and enable us to have enough clarity so that we will not compromise the therapy.

Some years ago, the International Association for Relational Psychoanalysis and Psychotherapy did a colloquium on "When the Frame Does Not Fit" by Anthony Bass. In that discussion, Paul Williams, a UK psychoanalyst, wrote that a patient's most profound disturbance is enacted through boundary violations. From this perspective, money provides a valuable boundary and, therefore, symbol by which we can often reach the deepest disturbances within our clients and, indeed, ourselves! In the following brief case study, I show how money featured in the psychotherapy.

A young Black British born, Afro-Caribbean man presented himself for therapy and seemed to expect me to lower my fee. Although I have a sliding scale, in this instance, I bristled at the feeling of his expectation that I would automatically lower my fee and intuitively held out against it. I did worry that he might think I was racist for not conforming to his view of how I should be as a white middle class psychotherapist, but I contained that feeling. I was glad I had done so when, several weeks later, while donning his new leather jacket, he told me he was off for a winter holiday in the sun for a few weeks, so would miss some sessions and he did not want to pay for them. Further, he mentioned that he was going with his brother, leaving his wife and their unborn child behind. I felt very irritated with him, but glad too, that I had not lowered my fee: it felt connected. At the same time, although I charge for missed sessions, I felt unable to ask him to do so and was aware that this was problematic on my behalf. My view was that it would be too much for him to bear psychologically to pay for something he was not actually receiving.

As the therapy progressed, I came to understand that he had had significant experience, both educationally and through his work, in the helping professions of white people rescuing him. His previous therapist, for example, had seen him for virtually no fee and, my client complained, seemed to want to talk about race all the time and how the client felt about the therapist's whiteness. I wondered if, in some strange way, these attitudes produce a re-enactment of the whole experience of slavery or apartheid—in this case by disinvesting my client of his responsibility for himself, his life, and so on. The issue of personal responsibility turned out to be central to this client's issues, which were about him becoming a father and his deep ambivalence, his lack of Black male role models, and his fear that he would lose his sexual identity which seemed to dominate his sense of self.

I think that psychological change was enabled to happen within the intersubjective domain of relatedness, in part, because he did not identify me as a white rescuing type, because of the position I took about the money. Indeed, he must have also sensed that I did not feel any urge to rescue him (in fact it was the opposite urge I had to deal with in my countertransference). I think these factors made it possible for him to transfer onto me in a very different way, which then offered him opportunities to find other types of, as yet, unknown self states.

One day, he told me that I was like Camilla Parker Bowles. Containing my lack of feeling flattered by this, I explored the meaning with him further and it seemed that this comparison meant that he found me to be intelligent, warm, and someone to whom he could say anything and feel understood. (We had talked lots about racism he was experiencing in his counsellor training group and had felt empowered by my analysis of the type of racism he was exposed to—often patronising and disempowering attitudes about Black men). But I still wondered about the introduction of the upper classes into our relationship. Lots of possible interpretations, of course, but I felt that there must be some meaning in this about "us," and that if I was Camilla, then maybe he was a Prince, a King in waiting. This made me notice his regal features. He was a beautiful man, with an aristocratic looking face. We began to wonder about his African ancestry and hypothesise about who and where he may have come from. I thoroughly enjoyed entering into the imaginative possibilities contained in his unknown past. There began to be a huge sense of uplifted self esteem, self motivation in the quality of our meetings, and with this came an increased sense of responsibility and a conscious desire to provide for, protect, and be responsible to his partner and unborn child.

So some questions for us to think about as psychotherapist:

1   How do our own Script issues impact upon the therapy?
2   How conscious are we of our own primitive fears about money?
3   How does money as a boundary operate in our own practices?
4   What is the effect if we cave in through a compassionate impulse to lower the fee?
5   What is the effect if we stick too rigidly to contracts around money?

REFLECTIONS

I was asked to offer a paper for the London-based Relational Psychoanalytic group on the subject of money. As usual, I turned to case material to demonstrate theory in action. My thoughts immediately turned to Charles. He was a young and very beautiful Black man who was in training at the Metanoia Institute to become a counsellor. I was interested in him because he said from our initial meeting, he really did not want to talk about race. In *The Multi Cultural Imagination*, Vannoy (1996) accesses the racial internal world and, in doing so, describes how white people can also be Black. This felt right to me because when I was born they thought I was Black; and that further, the hospital was being racist because all the Black babies were on one side of the ward. I channelled this part of me when working with Charles alongside my knowledge of African Caribbean history, in part from my work over five years at Brixton College. It was one of the most fascinating therapies I have ever done. We seemed to enter a "new world order" where Charles drew on his imagination to make me in to a Queen and himself into a King. We traced his ancestors to Ghana and together, in the room, we worked through his challenge to become the father of his unborn child from the perspective of a King, and not from his "other" history of enslavement where fathers were denied their legitimate role in the family, separated, and treated inhumanly.

Schore (1994) tells us the relational alliance happens though right-brain to right-brain connection. I did not use Charles to deal with my "white guilt" as did his former therapist. Indeed, I did not have any "white guilt"; but I was intellectually very well informed about racism. Instead of dealing with the hard facts of racism, I went along with my experience of him, his beauty, his sharp intellect, and his deep vulnerability. We moved into a metaphorical mythical place (McGilchrist, 2019) where transformation could happen through a subtle recalibration of affective regulation. The metaphor allowed his initial hostility to becoming a father to transform into a passionate advocate of fatherhood. We developed a mutual appreciation of each other as "royal personages," and examined how such royal personages come with ethical expectations of how to behave in the world—especially as a parent (even when they sometimes do not)!

Following the metaphor of king and queen, it felt like we had entered a cocreated play. I thought of *A Midsummer Night's Dream* in which metamorphosis occurs. People are altered and changed through the use of a love potion. As said, I found Charles beautiful and masterful, which was perhaps the equivalent of the "love potion" in *Midsummer Night's dream*; my insistence upon seeing him, not as a beggar, but as a beautiful young man refusing to offer him a reduced fee. This "love potion" had the effect of transforming both of us, out of our "ordinary clothes" into the higher realm of royalty. My refusal to lower my fee was directly linked to the royal metaphor we cocreated. From a beggar to a king in nine short months (the length of the therapy).

Chapter 13

The Erotic Relational Matrix Revisited

Helena Hargaden

The subject of erotic transference and countertransference is rarely addressed in our training, supervision or journals. In this article I propose that by underestimating the significance of these dynamics we are doing ourselves, our clients, and our profession, a considerable disservice. I begin this article with some personal experiences to highlight why the erotic seems to be so threatening. I set the erotic transference in its historical context, and, drawing on the work of Gabbard (1997), explore the most likely reasons for sexual transgressions. I conclude with the importance of recognising the inherent transformational potential of the erotic and finally suggest a model I have developed, based on relational methodology and techniques.

Personal, Clinical Experiences

I first became aware of erotic feelings in the therapeutic relationship when I had a dramatic dream, which informed me, or may be it would be more accurate to say *warned* me, that there were sexual feelings between me and my client whom I called Jonathon (Hargaden & Sills, 2002). Following on from this experience, I became interested in this type of transference and sought to promote a wider discussion on the topic within the TA world. I soon learned that any mention of the erotic in the professional domain arouses anxiety, shame, potential humiliation, and a sense of danger. Dimen (2003) describes it as the "'eew!' factor." For example when I introduced my paper, "There Ain't No Cure For Love" at the ITA Conference in Keele (Hargaden, 2001) with discussants Erskine (2001) and Sills (2001), the panel ended with some tittering in the audience and some attempts to make me feel uncomfortable. When this article was published in the *Transactional Analysis Journal*, Steiner (2003) attempted to redefine the clinical case misrepresenting it as an ordinary incidence of social "fancying" each other. I felt a strong invitation to feel embarrassed about my article and to consider that what I had written was perhaps rather silly. I found it helpful, in this context, to read Dimen (2003), who links shame and hatred with the emergence of the erotic. Her inspirational writing enabled me to understand the type of

DOI: 10.4324/9781032266237-14

uneasy dynamics I could sometimes find myself in when I attempted to open this discussion with my colleagues. It is not only the "eew" factor aroused in most people but also the extent of the collective disavowal of the erotic (Gabbard, 1997), which contributed to my sense of unease and the denial I encountered whenever I raised the topic. I think this collective disavowal costs us dear.

A few years after these publications about the erotic, a TA colleague told me that she had been privy to a discussion about them in which some transactional analysts had speculated that I must be talking about my unmet sexual needs. This is to miss the point. I was not getting my sexual needs met; besides the comment obviously came from a rather concrete and limited mind they had missed the fundamental issue that I was *acknowledging* my feelings. This is not enough in itself of course. The most significant thing I did was to *reflect* on the possible meanings of the erotic feelings. For example, I initially denied my feelings, which only came into my consciousness through the dream. When I did recognise the erotic feelings, I felt threatened by them. I wondered if I was a bad therapist because I found my client sexually attractive. When I began to realise that my feelings could be useful to the therapy, I started to ponder the significance of them and wonder about what my client might be trying to communicate to me through this unconscious process. Maybe there has been a fantasy contamination within the TA community that to describe the erotic makes it into a concrete act? Indeed it is far more likely that the opposite is the truth: analysis of countertransference feelings makes it more likely that the erotic feelings will stay in the realm of the symbolic and analytic space, and less likely that they will be acted out. It is when we misinterpret erotic feelings as concrete expressions to be repressed that we are most in danger of enactment. In the case referred to aforementioned Jonathon's deepest yearnings and needs emerged in our relationship. By acknowledging our sexual feelings, we explored his deepest fear that we would enact the feelings, which coupled with a strong hope that we would. There is a direct parallel here with incest in the family. The child seeks adoration, love, attunement, and, as we know, strokes of any sort, and because children are also sexual beings, sexuality is part of this. They may sit playfully on our knee, and even "turn us on," but our job is both to avoid rejecting or humiliating the child and to contain our own aroused desires. For a man, this is especially important if he has an erection (Blake-Morrison, 2001). Of course in the therapeutic situation, the fact that there is also another sexual adult in the room complicates our job even further. It is ridiculous to suggest that people who are having their sexual needs met will not experience the erotic in many other relationships and for it to have many meanings in these different relationships. Again it is to miss the point which in my case was that the client *needed* me to "fall in love" with him. Initially nothing could have been further from my thoughts or feelings as I had not found him remotely attractive and indeed had been rather repulsed by him. Interestingly, and significantly, it turned out that Jonathon's mother had been deeply depressed at his birth, in love with another man, not the father. It seemed that my client had never aroused that primal love, which also contains the erotic (Kraemer, 1999) and which he so cleverly, unconsciously elicited in me in order to move toward psychological health. Another way of understanding this process is to recognise that the client is attempting to find the "new, developmentally needed object in order to address a primitive longing" (Little, 2007, personal communication).

The Shadow of the Erotic

It is understandable that psychotherapists are instinctively and appropriately cautious of the erotic, which is why I am sympathetic to the defensive reactions that I have encountered. Nevertheless, in order to protect ourselves, our clients, and our profession, it is important to overcome our resistances, initially by acknowledging the significant role the erotic plays in our work. Knowledge gives us power and supports the developing maturity of the therapist, whereas denial keeps us in the primary school of neat circles, pretty colours where everything makes "sense," allowing us to remain youthful, naïve and even encourages stupidity. I know several cases where sexual transgressions have ended careers, damaged marriages, and generally wreaked havoc on peoples' lives. Guggenbuhl-Craig (1971) suggests that power is the shadow of the helping professions. When we deny the power contained in the erotic, it hovers in the shadows and comes out of the blue when we least expect it. Yet, as psychotherapists, we know that once we begin talking about the "forbidden," it loses some of its power over us. This power is not always for the ill; Mann (1999) describes the erotic as psychically binding bringing individuals into a deep relationship with each other. He proposes that both patient and therapist share unconscious erotic desires and suggests that the therapist aims to mediate these desires into what might be thought of as "good enough" incestuous desires. For those psychotherapists who are willing and able to enter relationships of depth with their clients, they need to be conscious of the erotic and know how to work with it.

Without this awareness, relational TA psychotherapists, at worst, are making themselves unnecessarily vulnerable, and at the very least, they could be missing signals that the client is striving toward psychological health, vitality, and growth that are often suggested by this type of transference. Moreover, it is arguable that those psychotherapists who stay in what appear to be the less risky waters of cognitive behavioural therapy are also at risk of enactment, maybe even more so, because of the tendency to work more with the concrete than the symbolic (see further).

History of the Erotic Countertransference

In his article, "Sexual Attraction and Phobic Dread in the counter-transference," Tansey (1994) tells us that the first documented erotic countertransference was the well-known analysis of Anna O by Breuer in 1880. Tansey describes how Breuer was obsessed by his beautiful young patient to the extent that his wife began to get jealous. Ending the treatment out of fear, his final session with Anna found her "confused and writhing with abdominal cramps" (p.142). She cried, "Now comes Dr. B's child" (p.142). It is not hard to imagine how terrifying this would have felt for Breuer and he left immediately, later referring her onto to another colleague. Breuer's is the first documented case of erotic transference and counter-transference although this was not how they saw it at the time. In the light of our collective disavowal of the erotic transference in psychotherapy, it is quite sobering, even amazing, to consider that this erotically charged therapeutic relationship launched the original talking cure, psychoanalysis, in 1880 with Breuer and Freud's book *Studies in Hysteria*. Freud's relationship with Jung was marred by Jung's sexual involvement with his patient Sabina Spielrein of which Freud disapproved. He attempted to dissuade Jung from his actions but to no avail. Writing to Jung in 1909 Freud uses the term "countertransference" for the first time, in relationship to Jung and Breuer's erotic enactments (Tansey, 1994, p. 143)

> Such experiences, *(in the countertrasnference),* though painful, are necessary and hard to avoid. Without them we cannot really know life and what we are dealing with. I myself have never been taken in quite so badly, but I have come very close to it a number of times and had a narrow escape. I believe that only grim necessities weighing on my work and the fact that I was ten years older than yourself when I came to psychoanalysis have saved me from such experiences. But no lasting harm is done. They help us to develop the thick skin we need and to dominate the "countertransference," which is after all a permanent problem for us; they teach us to displace our own affects to best advantage. They are a blessing in disguise. The way these women manage to charm us with every conceivable psychic perfection until they have attained their purpose is one of nature's greatest spectacles. (Freud quoted in Tansey).

Although Freud disapproved of Jung and later Ferenczi who married one of his patients, even he betrayed his principles when he encouraged a patient, one of his training analysts, to divorce his wife and marry his patient. The consequences were catastrophic for everyone, the wife died, the analyst became psychotic and the new marriage collapsed. Such disastrous conse-quences, including the break up of collegial relations, (Freud's break with

Breuer, Jung and Ferenczi were, amongst other matters, all connected to their erotic enactments), are one of the reasons why the erotic was repressed because it was seen as a very negative influence. It is also significant that Breuer, Freud, and Jung blame the women for what happens and do not take responsibility for their own actions.

It is difficult to find a history of the erotic in transactional analysis. Eric Berne's view was characteristically pragmatic. For instance, in *Games People Play* (1968) and in *Sex in Human Loving* (1973), he identifies the elements of seduction, guilt, hostility, excitement, pleasure, and other factors aroused by erotic situations. However, he tends to focus on a rational exposition of the psychological, social, and existential gains of such behaviour. Whilst this understanding is useful, it easily becomes defensive rather than containing for a therapist who has not explored her internal world sufficiently to hold and contain complex projections.

Cornell (2001) wrote a robust critique of my work, in which he drew our attention to contemporary thinking about hysteria and its origins in gender and sexuality. Drawing on the work of Bollas (2000), he requires us to revisit the subject of hysteria, avoiding the unconscious misogyny of Freud and Breuer, as a way of conceptualising some of the meanings that may be contained in the erotic transference and countertransference. Curiously little else has been written on the subject in TA journals or books since. The original article as well as the responses from the original discussants (Cornell, 2001; Erskine, 2001; Sills, 2001) provide an opportunity within transactional analysis to learn about the development of relational TA thinking as it pertains to the erotic (Cornell & Hargaden, 2005).

Sexual Transgressions

Gabbard's excellent work on this subject is mostly concentrated on psychoanalysts but is relevant for psychotherapists of whatever ilk. The conclusions he comes to make interesting reading for us all in the talking profession. For instance, most transgressions involve a male analyst and a female patient, about 20% of cases involve female therapists, and about 20% involve same-sex dyads.

Gabbard (1997, p. 2) argues that one of the primary ways the analytic profession deals with the phenomenon of therapy sexual abuse is through projective disavowal such as the following type of statements:

> Sexual boundary violations only occur in a small and marginal group of psychopathic analysts who have nothing in common with me.

Gabbard (ibid p. 2) says the facts are otherwise and that he has repeatedly received requests to evaluate people of whom has been said,

This is the last person we ever thought would be involved in an ethical transgression. He has been a pillar of the analytic community. He has been a valued teacher and supervisor of all of us.

Some people think the rules do not apply to them. They are "exceptions" who can get away with things that others cannot. Gabbard stresses certain life stressors, such as divorce, loss, and other personal misfortunes, any of us may become vulnerable to using patients as objects to gratify our emotional needs.

In one case that was brought to my attention, the therapist had allowed the boundaries to gradually be broken through email, mobile phone usage, and texting. According to Gabbard, virtually all sexual involvement between analyst and patient begins with subtle breaks in the frame that lead progressively to the final denouement.

Gabbard (ibid) distinguishes four areas in which therapists are most likely to enact out their sexual countertransference:

1   When the therapist is psychotic.
2   When the therapist has a predatory form of psychopathy and/or perversions.
3   When the therapist is lovesick.
4   When the therapist is involved in a masochistic surrender.

Psychosis is rare. Predatory psychopathy, which is also rare, describes a group that includes persons with severe narcissistic personality disorders. These therapists have a grandiose sense of entitlement, which "enables" them to exploit patients for their own needs. Recently I taught the erotic transference and countertransference. With a strange synchronicity, the following week, in the therapy group I run, the first client to speak told us that family friends had gone to therapy because their marriage was in trouble. He went onto say that the husband had stopped going and the wife had begun an affair with the therapist. Before I had a chance to respond, another man piped up to say that he too knew of a case where the therapist had apparently "fallen in love" with her client. He told us in a rather sarcastic tone that the client had been a wealthy man. Three other members then recounted personal experiences of when a therapist had behaved in a sexually suspicious way and betrayed their therapy. I had not said anything at this point and by the time they had all spoken, I was rather inclined to hide under my chair in embarrassment at the evidence of such pervasive misconduct in my profession. I was struck by the coincidence of these transgressions emerging in the therapy group so soon after my teaching the subject almost as if they had unconsciously picked up my receptivity to hearing about these transgressions. The reported incidents seemed to confirm Gabbard's assertion that sexual enactments were far more common than it was customary to acknowledge. I wondered too, in the case of the therapist and the wealthy client, if this might be one of the rare examples of psychopathy. Money has long been known for its aphrodisiac qualities and a cynical part of me can see how the therapist may have exploited her position to abuse her client in this way. I am not so sure training or supervision would make much difference to this group of therapists, which is depressing but at least realistic. Although it might be that training institutes need to be more rigorous in responding to narcissistic defences observed during a person's training, in order to protect the public (Little, 2007, personal communication).

Most of us will more easily recognise our vulnerability to be in the last two categories within which the majority of sexual transgressions take place. The lovesick group refer to those analysts who are in some type of life crisis, such as the illness of a child or spouse, the death of a family member, or profound marital problems. This group is inclined toward narcissistic injury rather than personality disorder. As we get older these life events become more likely and it is perhaps useful to consider our vulnerability to these issues and events while we are strong enough to think about how we may deal with it if the time ever comes. According to Gabbard (ibid p. 3), masochistic surrender describes the dynamic when therapists take pride in treating the so-called impossible or difficult patient.

> These analysts appear to pursue humiliation and victimisation in their work and often in their private lives as well. A common scenario involves a male analyst who is treating a female patient with a history of incest. The patient demands demonstrations of the analyst's caring, and the analyst uses reaction formation to defend against growing resentment and hatred towards the patient. The analyst attempts to demonstrate genuine "caring" for the patient (with an increasing disregard for professional boundaries) by holding the patient, extending the hour, and meeting the patient outside the office. They re-create an internal object relationship involving a tormentor and a tormented victim. This group of therapists distinguish themselves through their suffering and their willingness to "run the extra mile" with the patient.

I imagine some of us recognise elements of ourselves in this description maybe prior to deeper explorations in our personal therapy about why we have chosen and what we are doing in this profession. Many of us are probably familiar with clients who complain that we don't "care" enough, that because they pay it is not "real," and who make demands upon us to demonstrate our "genuineness." It may make us uncomfortable to feel the extent of our hostility toward someone who "deserves" compassion and we may resist knowing our real feelings while trying to keep a relational alliance with the client. A therapist can find himself in an untenable position, having broken boundaries and getting into deeper waters, until there feels to be a point of no return. Although these are exactly the dynamics Berne warns us about, I know of two cases where the therapist had thought he was protected by the "contract" and did not recognise what was happening to him until it was too late. The unconscious process had "tricked" the logical mind into a state of complacency because it thought it was in control.

One of the major causes of enactment is when the symbolic is understood in a concrete way. For example, when erotic feelings emerge, the therapist and the client may feel that the only way to deal with them is to act them out. Gabbard refers to this as a collapse of the analytic play space and argues that men in particular are vulnerable to this error of judgement. For instance psychotherapists will argue that "this is the real thing" and forget the transferential aspects of the relationship.

Transformational Potential

While this chapter focuses upon the betrayal of the erotic when this is acted upon and acted out, I want to acknowledge the power for good inherent in this transference when betrayal is avoided. Cornell puts the situation very well when he wonders if "we dance on a knife edge between disaster and possibility" (2001 p. 13).

What about the creative aspect of the erotic, in terms of life instinct and energy? Mann (1997) links the universality of the erotic unconscious to the presence of incestuous desire. He proposes that both patient and therapist share unconscious erotic desires and suggests that the therapist aims to mediate these desires into what might be thought of as "good enough" incestuous desires. It is arguable that a therapy, which does not acknowledge the erotic, is also damaging to the client. Samuels (1999) believes that if the therapist/analyst has anything to offer by definition it will be dangerous. My intuitive sense is that people often come into therapy feeling bad about themselves and that it is only love that can change this around. From this perspective, the question is not whether we feel erotic love for a client but rather why don't we feel this love in relation to a particular client? Tudor (personal communication, 2007) points out that in ancient Greek, whose language is generally more nuanced than English, there are four words that describe different kinds of love: agape (self-giving), philia (friendship), epithymia (sexual desire), and Eros, meaning the quest for fulfilment. This makes clear the important of the erotic in relationship; indeed one may say that by definition, relationship is erotic.

This subject raises our deepest fears and because of this, we need to feel contained theoretically. I propose the following model as a guide for the clinician to work with the erotic transference. This model is grounded in TA literature on the transferential relationship including Moiso (1984), Novellino (1984/1990), Hargaden and Sills, (2002), and Little (2006). The model also relies upon a willingness by the therapist to engage with in-depth psychotherapy so that she is not a stranger to her own desires, yearnings, and needs and how this emerges in her own therapy.

Relational Methodology and Technique

Drawing on Benjamin's 22 principles of relational psychoanalysis (2002), I identify the central features of Relational TA methodology (Hargaden, 2007; in press) as follows:

The crucial significance of relationship

Therapy as a two-way street involving a bi directional process

The vulnerability of therapist and client

Counter-transference is used, not only as information but possibly in thoughtful disclosure and mutual dialogue

The co-construction and multiplicity of meaning

The relational unconscious

Intuitive use of techniques

The following model identifies the type of techniques to consider when thinking about the erotic transference:

An acknowledgement of the existence of erotic feelings
Through use of associations, dreams, and an analysis of our emotional and behavioural responses to our clients, we can begin to recognise any elements of the erotic in our countertransference.

An analysis and reflection of countertransference for possible meanings
It is important to learn to play with possibilities, and not to get fixed on just one meaning.

A distinction between the erotic as an attack on the relationship and the erotic as a means toward transformation.
These are not mutually exclusive processes but sometimes the client may try to sexualise the therapy as a way of avoiding emotional connection. This will be experienced as a narcissistic attack on relationship (Little, 2006) rather than an attempt to emotionally connect.

An appreciation of the erotic as symbolic
It is important to recognise the erotic as symbolic and not concrete. When a therapist starts to give her clients objects, to speak with the client outside of the therapy hour, or to accept clients' comments as concrete expressions without any attempt at interpretations she could be heading toward trouble!

An understanding of projective identification and inter-penetration (bidirectionality).
In matters of the erotic, it is very useful to have an understanding of this type of transference. It is quite possible to feel "taken over" through this type of unconscious dynamic. Indeed, "falling in love" could be said to be a projective, inter-penetrative experience. We are hopefully all familiar with the sensations associated with this process. It can feel as though one is in a delirious state of being, fevered, with rapid heart-beats, a dry mouth, and a feeling that one has been taken over by one's deepest yearnings and longings. This state amounts to an alteration of consciousness in which our usual judgements are skewed. Yet we may convince ourselves that we are completely Adult and thinking sensibly. It is essential to understand this type of projective identification and seek help through consultation immediately. The novel and recent film *Notes on a Scandal* (2006) demonstrates this process very well, in which a young female teacher loses all sense of appropriateness and is literally "taken over" by the senses and desires of not only her self but also the other, in a love which is shown to be fundamentally exploitative on both sides.

The use of self disclosure.
The question here is how to engage with these issues in a sensitive manner. How do we translate our countertransference into an emotionally connecting and relevant transaction? It may be that we alter our attitude or behaviour in some subtle way or it may be necessary to raise the matter verbally. In the case where I had my dream, I said to the client, "I think there are sexual feelings between us," I later discovered that by finding a way to refer to my countertransference, I intuitively enabled us to make the sexual feelings in the dream into what Ogden (1991) calls an object of knowledge for reflection. In this instance, my self disclosure meant the client was able to reflect on the feelings and come to recognise that he could feel both affection and sexual feelings with the same person. Until then his sexuality had been expressed in a Madonna-v-whore type split.

A particular question arises about disclosure when it is a male therapist with a female client. How do they reflect matters of sex and sexuality in a way which is not gratuitous on the one hand, yet shows they are taking the feelings seriously on the other? When a female client referred to something "down there," the male therapist knew it was significant but was also terribly conscious of the shaming aspect of this. He was able to deal with it in a very sensitive way, without ignoring it; he picked up her confusion and shame and responded to it empathically while offering her the sensitive interpretation that she wished to explore something sexual with him and at the same time this felt frightening and shameful. As therapists, we must always be asking ourselves the question of how to have a conversation about these things. We need to bear in mind too the client's state of mind. A client in a concrete state of mind, functioning at a primitive level, may hear our interpretation or comments, not as a metaphor, but as an intention. The question here is: when and how to say something and perhaps when to delay saying something (Little, 2007, personal communication).

The use of the erotic to trace the evolution and development of the therapeutic relationship.
Sometimes it feels like the erotic has you in its "grip." For example, I was alerted to the developmental needs inherent in the erotic when, in my dream, I dreamt the client was leaning over to give me a kiss in an erotically charged moment, only to morph into an 18-month-old baby at the point of contact. When a client stares at us adoringly, and tells us all about their life, without wanting too much input from us, we can recognise the idealised transference and know that the therapy is in its early stages. Guntrip (1962) said that as he drew toward the end of each analysis, he experienced warmth and affectionate feelings toward his patient and would happily have married them (men or women). This feels to me to be a useful measurement of knowing when therapy is moving toward its end because there is a sense of a more mature type of love, where there is mutual respect, affection, liking, and closeness, which can often include sexual feelings in the knowledge, sometimes sadly, that nothing will ever happen between you.

A contemporary understanding of the Oedipus Complex
Freud drew on the Sophocles myth of Oedipus in order to understand incestuous longings. He has been criticised about this for, among other things, using it to disguise the fact that his patients had been sexually abused by their fathers Masson, (1988/19990). However revisiting the Oedipus complex from a contemporary perspective (Britton, 1998; Mann, 1997) clinicians may find it useful to consider several aspects of the Oedipal complex when working with the erotic.

Perhaps the most important aspect is to consider the significance of the "third" in the psychological development toward maturity. Traditionally, this was thought to be the "father" but contemporary thinkers (Aron, 2006) interpret the "third" as anything, which forces the child/client to recognise that he or she not the sole focus of the mother/therapist's benevolent attention. This recognition is essential if the client is to be helped to individuate from an idealised notion of mother. Britton (1998) describes how his patient cries out to him, "Stop that fucking thinking."

His patient feels abandoned by the therapist because the therapist is involved with his own internal object, which represents a type of "third" in the relationship, as when the mother has a relationship with the father, the analyst is having a relationship in his head. In this example, thinking is an oedipal object; it is like an internal intercourse. This view challenges a relational sense that we should always be "attuned" to our clients and "available" to hear their every word, which of course creates a rather contrived relationship. At some point, in order to grow, the client needs to recognise the therapist's separateness. This can be very difficult for some clients who have deeper narcissistic injuries than others. For example, when I broke my foot last year, thereby bringing indisputable evidence of my vulnerable and separate self into therapeutic relationships, one client sat in such a way as to avoid seeing my plaster cast. It was an oedipal object. Our reflections on this "intrusion" into the therapy have raised the painful consciousness of how much the client had denied my separateness and of the resistance to psychological growth contained in that denial.

I have concentrated on the therapeutic relationship in this discussion but all relationships that are inherently asymmetrical such as the training and supervisory relationships can also emerge these dynamics and again discussion seems taboo (Napper, 2007, personal communication). It would be odd indeed if most, if not all, of our relationships did not hold aspects of the erotic. Gerrard, in her lovely article, asks her therapist the following question, recounting the therapist's oh so wise response:

"When will I know that you love me?"

"When you come to feel loved by me, then you will know."

(Gerrard, 1999 p. 29)

REFLECTIONS

I wrote this chapter out of a feeling of frustration and wanting myself and the community to grasp the dangers inherent in our work. As psychotherapists, we offer ourselves up in so many ways. We pledge ourselves to others. We listen attentively, reflectively, and we talk our meditations through with our therapists and supervisors. Nevertheless our profession is plagued by errors of judgement when therapists falls foul of the ethics of our profession. It is a two-way street. Some people come to us and our analytic love is not enough. They want our soul. The therapist, as explained in the chapter, may also find that analytic love is not enough and they want the soul of the client. Soul connection. Soul lovers. When enacted, soul murder. I have at times felt strongly drawn into a "love" connection with some clients, a "love" connection that could feel extraordinary and even wonderful if it could only be sexual. This is what makes our profession so ethically tricky and potentially dangerous. I recall a woman came to see me and I had two visceral responses of her in about 60 seconds. I felt connected with her, warm and loving and as she sat down and began speaking I felt repulsed and disgusted. This process was validated when she told me how she had slept with her former therapist. My feeling response was one of empathy for the therapist she had managed to lure him into what felt like her web of destruction. Nevertheless, no matter how we may spin it, it is entirely up to the therapist to keep the sexual boundary.

Chapter 14

Then We'll Come from the Shadows

Helena Hargaden

In this chapter, I present my keynote speech given at the Southeast Transactional Analysis conference in Tunbridge Wells, Kent, England, in June 2003. The conference was organised by Mark Head and supported by Joanna Beazley-Richards and Stephen Richards from Wealdon College. The theme was "Developing Transactional Analysis."

When asked to deliver this keynote address, I found my thoughts wandering toward Eric Berne and how, if he had not existed and used his genius to create TA, none of us would exist as transactional analysts today. This led me to think about how Berne is our TA "father"; and then I began to wonder who he was and what he was really about. I remembered that he had changed his name from Bernstein to Berne, something I have often vaguely wondered about in terms of its meaning.

I decided that this was the question I wanted to consider today: What impact did changing his name from Bernstein to Berne have on him and, subsequently, on TA theory? I think this provides an interesting way to begin to pick apart our TA script, to understand our TA parent, and to analyse our games, rackets, and so on. This is, after all, what we do with ourselves and our clients. To understand ourselves better, we look at our fore bearers and try to understand where we came from and what made us who we are. From this process, we often find new, creative parts of ourselves. I would like to see if we can do this with Berne and TA, in order to understand our forefather better, unpick our TA script, and find creative parts of ourselves as transactional analysts.

What was Berne really like? Although I have read his works, Ian Stewart's (1992) book on Eric Berne, and the Jorgensens' (1984) biography; and have heard things about him over the years, I still, somehow, did not really have a sense of him or feel any natural empathy toward him. He was just a man with glasses, with a dry wit, who was very talented and had developed a clever theoretical model. I thought it a shame that I could find no feelings for him. This prompted me to consider what it must have been like for a young Jewish man growing up in Canada in the 1930s and 1940s—to imaginatively put myself in his shoes. I

DOI: 10.4324/9781032266237-15

remembered how, in 1943, while Berne was living in New York and training to be a psychoanalyst, he changed his name from Bernstein (pronounced "-steen") to Berne. He later wrote, "The choice is whether to keep the name and make it illustrious like the conductor, Leonard Bernstein (steyn) or to change it altogether and turn one's back on the Semitic factor" (Jorgensen & Jorgensen 1984, p. 34).

Now the background is that Jews often changed their names. I learned that there is a Rabbinic principle dating back to 200 BC whereby if you recovered from a serious illness, had done something terrible, or were about to die, you could change your name and symbolically become another person. That is, there is a type of spiritual license to change one's name; it is meant to be a transformational process. But the principle has also become perverted so that people change names to belong with the perceived "winners" of society. Was Berne's change a transformational process or a perverted one? I think it was both. It seems clear that he did it to move away from being seen as a Victim, that he gave up his Semitism so that he could make it (although he never did) and control how people saw him. However, in giving up his Semitism, he never had to directly confront his victimhood, and thus attempted to move away from the shameful feelings attached to being a victim.

There is no doubt that changing his name made Berne less vulnerable. When he did it in 1943, three thousand people a day were being exterminated in the gas chambers of Nazi Germany. And in Vichy France, many French Jews, who had previously considered themselves French citizens, had been betrayed by that government and handed over to the Nazis to perish in the camps. Jews worldwide were learning that no matter how well they had done or how much they thought they belonged to and had integrated themselves into the countries of their birth, that they were, first and foremost, Jewish people who were despised, hated, and hunted. So, as Berne was seeking US citizenship, he must have felt lucky to be alive and unsure as to how welcome he would be as a Jew. In fact, many people in the world were shocked to realise the extent of the Holocaust and the extermination camps, and maybe part of their shock was over what we as human beings are capable of. Putting Berne into the socioeconomic and historical context of his life allows us to understand him as a vulnerable, insecure, even fearful person. In leaving the "stein" behind, he clearly sought to make himself less vulnerable.

As a child in Montreal, Berne had experienced racial hatred from anti-Semitic children who spat on him on his way to school. Such exclusion breeds self-hatred. In addition, Berne was regularly beaten as a child by his father. Berne hated his hair and its tight curls because he thought it made him look too Jewish. There is certainly ample evidence in the Jorgensens' (1984) biography of the subtle and less subtle anti-Semitism to which Berne was exposed. This is most graphically demonstrated through the eyes of his first wife. A pretty, blonde, American gentile called Elinor, who, according to the Jorgensens, represented to Berne a means of emancipation from his constricted past; she was "everything he wanted to escape from the stigma of being a Jew, everything he wanted in a wife" (p. 28). Some time after Berne's death, Elinor said,

> Now I grieve for him. This was a kid who became convinced early in life that no one was ever going to love him. But he was going to dominate others through sheer brains and will, as if he were saying: I'll show them who has power!
>
> (Jorgensen & Jorgensen 1984, p. 29)

Clearly, our TA father felt too vulnerable and too conscious of his mortality to show his full self, and perhaps this contributed to why Berne's analysis was deemed incomplete and why he was never granted membership in his psychoanalytic institute. Although he often claimed that he was kicked out of the institute because of his unorthodox ideas, the Jorgensens' (1984) quoted a Dr. H. as saying,

> Somebody put out a story that Berne was kicked out of the Institute because of his unorthodox ideas. I don't know who could have put out such a story if it weren't Berne himself. But it wasn't true. I don't think Berne was kicked out because of non-adherence to dogma, unorthodoxy, or not sticking to the party-line. My feeling is that it was because of the severity of Berne's personal problems. (p. 154)

Maybe Berne could just not trust enough to enter fully into the analytic process, and maybe his therapy was incomplete. It is also possible that the establishment did not welcome his democratisation of the process of analysis. Berne was, indeed, a deeply wounded man; but if he had not been, perhaps he would not have created TA.

So, to return to my original question, what is the significance of the loss of "stein" for Berne? Could it be symbolic of the most vulnerable part of Berne, the hated, hunted, and despised part? We can understand this in script terms as Don't Feel, Don't Be You, and Don't Trust. From his father, he had the messages to look after his mother and sisters, to please and take care of others, and to be strong. The cultural script is clear as well: Don't Be You, it's too frightening; Don't Exist as you. If we take this unconscious script to its logical conclusion, could it be: Be strong; it's not safe to be who you are; you could be exterminated because you are vulnerable; you are other; you are despised, hunted, hated, not wanted. In changing his name, was Berne unconsciously seeking to deny, to get rid of, his vulnerability?

Berne's response to his rejection by the psychoanalytic community and his own analysis was to develop a theory that enabled people to take control, at least this was his declared goal as described by Stewart (1992):

> The goal of psychotherapy for Berne was not simply insight. Instead, psychotherapist and client should move assertively to bring about change and cure: The key to both is knowing how to act rather than knowing words. This stance represents a bold departure by Berne from the insight-oriented tradition of psychoanalysis. (p. 4)

Berne's emphasis was on taking the most pragmatic route, removing the splinter from the wound, taking action not using words. However, the ulterior message of such goals was to avoid, as much as possible, any vulnerability by working for declared objectives, aims, and control. Berne's theory reflected his own dilemma; he wanted someone to take the splinter out of his wound so he did not have to feel the pain. The splinter is an archetypal symbol for the hurts and wounds, and Berne wanted a theory that could rid us of those hurts without having to feel the hurt, the pain, the shame; without having to feel one's humanness. Fanita English observed to Berne,

> With dismay I often saw you operate with a rather callow sense of humour and sarcastic invitations for negative strokes. I now interpret these as substitutes which appeared whenever emotions related to neediness or softness or warmth threatened to surface. I see you as the skinny little Jewish kid with thick glasses and a big nose trying to make it in a Canadian grade school where boys were probably encouraged to have a stiff upper lip.
>
> (Jorgensen & Jorgensen 1984, p. 154)

This is a survival script, often a male script in particular, where softness, vulnerability, sentiment, and warmth (often qualities, however erroneously, associated with femininity) are treated with contempt and hate. We could describe it as a macho script or at the least a script that overemphasises the stereotypical masculine qualities of brains and brawn, external achievements, and material success, and that requires a denial of qualities such as warmth, neediness, and vulnerability, which are deemed inferior. This script not only applies to the Jews, a subject that has been thoroughly researched, but, also, I think, to any group that has suffered exclusion because of race, sexual orientation, religion, and so on. I propose that this enactment in our human drama, which we see and experience daily, reflects ambivalence about owning a part of our own psyches. It is as if a part of the psyche is continually denied, hated, and despised, and must be colonised, taken over, excluded, repressed, and even murdered.

No wonder, then, that Berne tried to leave "stein" behind—not only in his name but in his theory. First and foremost, Berne was angry with the establishment, as well he might be. On some level, he must have felt deeply angry about the way he had been treated by his father, his culture, and his adopted country. And this anger he used creatively to develop the theory of TA. He saw himself as a type of hero of the people, setting out to popularise analysis, debunk the mystique of the professionals, and give power to the people. This was an honourable aim, and in many ways he was successful. But an ulterior motive was to help people avoid misery through the use of contractual psychotherapy. It does not take much of an imaginative leap to realise how emphasising measurable contracts can lead to denying the existence of the contents of the vulnerable self and, in so doing, to make TA into a type of happy pill and to promote the insidious lie that it is never too late to have a happy childhood!

I think the ulterior result of this legacy is that TA as a theory, and maybe as an organisation, is often in denial of its shadow. And embedded within this denial of our shadow is a fear of the unconscious. After all, the underlying theme of transactional analytic concepts is to gain Adult control over our injuries and wounds as played out through games, rackets, and so on. However, what this often leads to is an overemphasis on the external world and achieving success in an external sense. What we lose is an understanding of the internal world; we are too hurried, too brusque, too knowing, and while our focus is on the external, on the light, we can too easily lose sight of the existence and significance of the interior world of our clients and of ourselves. In creating his theory, Berne sought to leave the world of "stein" behind and, in doing so, became separated from his unconscious and created a lopsided theory that contains within it a fear of what is not readily comprehensible, concrete, tangible, and, therefore, controllable.

From Berne's amazing theoretical concepts, we may be able to understand how we are heading for a breakdown but we cannot stop it, not always, not entirely. Out of Berne's genius, we find his vulnerability, and isn't that something to talk about? After all, isn't that the very essence of who we are, our humanness? At our most vulnerable, we may feel not wanted, not loved, desolate, full of loss and fear. Who has not felt these feelings? Why do we have to run away from them? However, if this is the case, then we cannot control what happens, we cannot live our life by contracts, outcomes, and socially controlled constructs. Once we recognise our true vulnerability, then we move into a very different land—the land of shadows—a land that Berne was frightened of, the land of "stein," of uncertainty, of the unknown, of possibility, of monsters and goblins, the land some may describe as the feminine. It is a too-often derided and devalued part of our world, psyche, selves, and culture, a part that we cannot quite grab hold of and control no matter how hard we try, a part of ourselves that comes up and strikes us out of the blue and reveals to us things about ourselves that we are frightened of, that remind us too much of a vulnerability that we would rather control.

Let us look at this feminine side, at this unexplored continent of the psyche symbolised by the moon with its bright and dark sides, at how exciting it is to be not controlled, to be not nurtured out of existence, to be freed to really think our own thoughts and feel our own feelings! The feminine, the relational, the connectedness, the loving, the human, the birthing, the giving, the tenderness—but let us not ignore the dark side, the envy, the controlling, and so on. But now we are faced with a paradox. Just as we berate our parents for getting it wrong, and in some cases much, much worse, we would not have a life without them and we can never thank them enough for that. So too with Eric Berne: He gave us life as transactional analysts.

To once again quote Fanita English,

> What I feel we should emphasise is that as a result of this man's influence, important changes took place in individuals and in society. That Eric dared and sometimes dared clumsily and stupidly, and out of his own compulsions (not always necessarily because of Adult decisions). It may be that, thanks to his crazy, compulsive daring, some of us did things and changed situations, systems, people, in a way that couldn't have been done otherwise. I want you to say this, not only from the perspective of "Oh, Eric was so wonderful!" but also from the perspective of someone like me who occasionally said, "Damn the guy!" Sometimes he was a bastard! He may have irritated people; he irritated me. However, without him hundreds of thousands of people would not have benefitted from what he had to teach.
>
> (Jorgensen & Jorgensen 1984, p. 38)

I think it is time for us to unite, to come from the shadows, to put the "stein" back into TA, to allow ourselves to learn that, paradoxically, the shadow is our most valued part. I think some of us are looking now to develop a theory that will allow for vulnerability, for acknowledging the despised part of the self, the part that is hunted, the part that will make us vulnerable. After all, one of the reasons why the Jews were slaughtered in Europe was because the Nazis projected their shadow onto them and then tried to rid themselves of it by murdering every last one.

I want to finish with the chorus from Leonard Cohen's song/poem entitled "*The Partisan*," which was about the French resistance to the Nazis: "Oh the wind the wind is blowing / through the graves the wind is blowing / freedom soon must come / then we shall come from the shadows."

REFLECTIONS

In Jungian analysis, at the time, I was fascinated by the idea of the shadow. The shadow part of our personality contains those things that we do not wish to be. I was curious about the shadow in Eric Berne and described his life experience in this talk. It reads as a critique of his work in which he placed great value on being a "winner." This goal disguised the fact that, in reality, he experienced himself as a "loser." This was not surprising, given his life experiences of anti Semitism. I was curious to examine how his state of mind affected the theory of TA in which he moved further away from his roots in psychoanalysis toward a cognitive behavioural paradigm that sought to "cure" people as quickly as possible. When I read this at a conference, I was moved and delighted to see one of the owners of a TA institute cry. It felt like a validation of a truth that our organisation does not want to own.

The relational approach seeks out new and unknown experience. Classical TA, developed by Berne, became increasingly routine, familiar, and the information gathered becomes the concern of the left hemisphere only (McGilchrist, 2009). So, intuition, feelings, new experiences, become less relevant. Berne initially placed heavy emphasis upon intuition but this concept quickly became shackled to evidence and was not allowed to stray too far from the models of TA he and others devised. Trainees were encouraged to see themselves and clients through the prism of TA theory. So a TA therapist might "know" a lot of information about themselves and their clients; but how to "know" someone from your experience of them is an entirely different matter (McGilchrist, ibid). From this perspective, diagnosis can describe a client in technical terms but it cannot capture the spirit, soul, and life of someone.

As depth psychotherapists, it is imperative that we examine our shadow. We all have a shadow and when we illuminate our shadow, something else of us moves into the shadow. To have no shadow would mean we were not alive. The shadow, therefore, is a significant part of who we are; and Berne's shadow throws light upon our understanding of his theory, his modis operandi, and leads to a feeling of warmth toward him but not an undying loyalty. Taking time to think about Berne's shadow can release us from the imperative to follow his thinking to stay only within the left-hemisphere and to mostly ignore other types of knowledge.

Chapter 15

The Irish Uprising of Easter 1916

A Psychopolitical Dialogue

Helena Hargaden and Keith Tudor

April 2016 marked the 100th anniversary of the Easter Rising in Ireland, which took place 24th–29th April 1916, predominantly in Dublin. Like any political event of this nature, the Easter Uprising demands a complex political, sociological, and psychological analysis; the present chapter offers subjective reflections on this event and its implications, and includes a number of historical and psychological references for the curious reader to deepen their understanding of this event for themselves.

The Historical

Organised by the Military Council of the Irish Republican Brotherhood (IRB), the Rising began on Easter Monday, 24th April 1916 and lasted for six days. The IRB was joined by members of the Irish Volunteers, the Irish Citizen Army, and Cumann na mBan (see Box 15.1), seized key locations in Dublin, and proclaimed an Irish Republic. Following the suppression of the Uprising, and trial under court martial all seven signatories to the Proclamation (see Box 15.1) were executed by firing squad.

The Personal

Helena: My grandmother lived in Francis Street, Dublin, in an area called "The Liberties" and I have since figured out that she must have met my grandfather when he "policed" the area, after 1916, to secure the peace. He was handsome man, black hair, green eyes, and she was known as a beauty, auburn hair and the bluest of eyes or so the story goes. They must have fallen in love, despite being on opposite sides of the "divide." They went off to live in Bray in County Wicklow, but, subsequent to the 1916 Uprising, my grandfather, who was originally from County Leitrim, was thought of as a traitor by his compatriots. They lived next door to the barracks of the Royal Irish Constabulary (RIC), with the

DOI: 10.4324/9781032266237-16

Box 15.1   The key organisations and Irish protagonists of the Easter Rising 1916

The Irish Republican Brotherhood (IRB) was a secret and aoth-bound organisation, established in 1858, dedicated to the establishment of an "independent democratic Ireland."

The Irish Volunteers (IV), or the Irish Volunteer Force or Irish Volunteer Army, was a military organisation established in 1913 by Irish nationalists in response to the formation of the Ulster Volunteers in 1912. Its primary aim was "to secure and maintain the rights and liberties common to the whole people of Ireland." Its leaders were Eoin MacNeill and Éamon de Valera.

The Irish Citizen Army was a small group of trained trades union volunteers from the Irish Transport and General Workers' Union, founded by James Larkin, James Connolly, and Captain Jack White.

Cumann na mBan (the Irishwomen's Council) was an Irish Republican women's paramilitary organisation formed in 1914.

The Key Irish Protagonists

Thomas James "Tom" Clarke, a republican, a member of the IRB, and, arguably, the person most responsible for the Easter Rising.

Seán Mac Diarmada, a political activist and revolutionary leader, a member of many associations which promoted the Irish language, Gaelic revival, and Irish nationalism; a close colleague and friend of Tom Clarke's.

Thomas MacDonagh, a political activist, poet, playwright, educationalist, and member of the Gaelic League; founding member of and Commandant of the 2nd Battalion, Dublin Brigade, of the Irish Volunteers.

Patrick Pearse, a teacher, barrister, poet, nationalist, and political activist, a member of both the IRB and the IV; the main voice of the Rising and idolised by Irish nationalists, his writings and reputation have been subject to some criticism on the basis of his fanaticism and religiosity.

Éamonn Ceannt, republican, member of the Gaelic League and the IRB; Commandant of the 4th Battalion, Dublin Brigade, of the Irish Volunteers.

James Connolly, a republican, socialist, and a leading Marxist theorist of his day.

Joseph Plunkett, a nationalist poet and journalist; one of the original members of the IRB military committee and primarily responsible for planning the Rising.

new incumbents of Black and Tans (a force of temporary con-
stables recruited to assist the RIC, the brainchild of Winston
Churchill then British Secretary for War), who were consistently
under attack by the Irish Republican Army (IRA). Bullet holes
were still to be found in their house when I first went there in the
1960s. You can imagine how this caused my grandmother to go
mad and my grandfather, an Irish man, born and bred in the West
country, to die of pernicious anemia at the age of 50. To me it
seems as though he died of a broken heart. My father was born
around 1923 into this dysfunctional, terrified, confused, split,
system.

Keith: I remember my mother, who was born in Downpatrick, Northern
Ireland, in October 1917, telling us of her childhood memories
of a house on fire, and a lot of noise and upset. I wonder about
how her father, my grandfather, a Unitarian minister and, by all
accounts, a quiet and gentle man, fared in the atmosphere of
religious and political sectarianism in which his peers would more
than likely have included some fairly fierce Protestant ministers.
As one of the peer reviewers of this chapter confirmed, the whole
place would have been fierce as Downpatrick is a kind of border
between Protestant North Down and Catholic South Down, and
has two cathedrals, one Anglican, one Catholic, facing each other
on adjacent hills.

Fast forward to the early 1980s when I was a very active political activist
and would often end the week in one of the Irish pubs in Hammersmith,
London, usually watching an Irish band who would always end the evening playing "Amhrán na bhFiann," the Irish national anthem. Whatever
the state of the debate or however many pints of Guinness had been
drunk, the whole pub would stand and sing. Depending on the news and
the state of the struggle, especially with regard to the Hunger Strikes of
1980 and 1981, there would often be anger in our hearts and tears in our
eyes. After all, this was only 15 years since the *Race Relations Act 1965*
had made it illegal to put up notices that had been standard in the West
London rented housing market: "No Blacks, no Irish, no Dogs." While
the notices had disappeared, the sentiment lingered. The English version
of the Irish anthem, The Soldiers' Song, had been used as a marching song
by the Irish Volunteers and by the "rebels" in the General Post Office in
Dublin during the Easter Rising of 1916. At the time I was living in a
collective house, which included two Irish women, whose politics and
experiences—including, at times and in certain situations, being fearful
of speaking as their accents would reveal their nationality—very much
influenced me.

Helena: Like you, I became involved in left wing politics, and joined the International Marxist Group (IMG), because, from my perception, they seemed to be the only Left wing group who understood, or were interested in "the Irish Question," which, by the 1970s, had become the dreadful Troubles. I sang rebel songs on the dock road folk clubs in Liverpool and was received enthusiastically by lovely people, who were very political, well meaning, with good intentions, but I always felt that they didn't quite "get it." I still am unsure of what that means, except that I was permanently in my feelings of things while they seemed very much in the intellect of things. Looking back, I think I was unconsciously carrying the weight of my father's grief, and his own father's grief and loss of being Irish because he had somehow, inadvertently, been on the "wrong side." I have spent 30 years in analysis of different types mostly dealing with this turbulent legacy and transgenerational trauma: of betrayals, loss, divisions, and nationalistic fervour and its impact on my Irish family. I now can understand how I was enacting the sense of being on "the wrong side" of being the "outsider."

Keith: I am struck by the symbolism of your grandfather policing an area called "The Liberties," and perhaps finding some liberty or liberation in doing so! It seems to me that there is an important dialectic between policing and liberty. Does policing always compromise or constrain liberty, or does liberty sometimes need the protection of the police? The name "The Liberties" dates back to the 13th century when certain areas within Dublin had their own jurisdiction, a meaning that echoes and evokes the sense of autonomy and liberty.

There is also a poignant theme of division and divisiveness and, of course, this is embodied in the political division of the geographical island of Ireland. One of my favourite rebel songs is—or was—"Four Green Fields" in which a mother weeps for the loss of one of her children/fields, that is, the province of Ulster:

"What did I have?" said the fine old woman
"What did I have?" this proud old woman did say.
"I had four green fields, each one was a jewel
But strangers came and tried to take them from me.
I had fine strong sons, they fought to save my jewels
They fought and died, and that was my grief" said she.
"Long time ago" said the fine old woman
"Long time ago" this proud old woman did say.
"There was war and death, plundering and pillage

My children starved by mountain valley and sea.
And their wailing cries, they shook the very heavens
My four green fields ran red with their blood" said she.

"What have I now?" said the fine old woman
"What have I now?" this proud old woman did say.
"I have four green fields, one of them's in bondage
In stranger's hands, that tried to take it from me.
But my sons have sons, as brave as were their fathers
My fourth green field will bloom once again" said she.

(Makem, 1967)

By the way, I don't agree about the IMG being the only group on the Left interested in the Irish Question. In the late 1970s and early 1980s, I was a member of Big Flame, a revolutionary socialist group (see https://bigflameuk. wordpress.com/about/) which, from its inception in 1975, expressed its unequivocal and uncritical support for Irish republican and revolutionary demands including (British) Troops Out and self-determination for the Irish people as a whole, that is, in all 32 counties.

And The Political

Helena: Yes, I do understand what you say about Big Flame. My recollection is that it was/you were also very interested in the Irish question, and, unlike some of the more dogmatic Left, more open in their thinking, but for many on the Left at that time Ireland was too close to home. They preferred struggles happening in far flung places such as those in Chile and Nicaragua about and for which they could voice their outrage and support, without drawing attention to themselves as potential allies of the IRA and thereby excite the interest of the Special Branch.

I, too, was drawn to Left wing groups in part because they embraced a type of romanticism about revolutions in general. Revolutions were considered to be a good thing. This made me feel proud about the Irish revolution. It was as if I had a revolution to boast about in my own back yard, so to speak! In those days revolution was in the air. We were young. We celebrated all and any revolution, didn't we? Perhaps revolutionary movements are essentially a young person's activity, a desire to kill the father as Freud (1913/1985) suggested, a Free Child expression of fearless energy as Berne might have said, or, an urge to transform, to make different through a type of collective projective identification, which, elsewhere, I have described as "transformational transference," meaning a process of deep psychological change through which consciousness can emerge (Hargaden & Sills, 2002). However, with the benefit of hindsight—and insight—through greater knowledge and maturity, I think and feel quite differently from those days in the IMG. I can see that my "activism" was mostly a personal expression of deep discontent and unhappiness rooted in trans-generational trauma, which was linked to the Troubles but in a deeply personal and slightly dissociated way. In today's environment I would not refer to myself as an activist. Romanticism is easy to come by; hard facts, complexity, and paradox all generate and require a more demanding and maybe quieter view of things.

For instance, thinking about Four Green Fields, which I also used to sing, my question now is: are these lyrics too rooted in the rhetoric of Romantic nationalism, with its themes of sacrifice and heroism? Do these sons of sons have to be as "brave as were their fathers," many of whom were killed? Patrick Pearce in particular extolled a puritanical idealisation of suffering as blood sacrifice. In this sense, the song simplifies this struggle by making it into a blood sacrifice as a way to gain unity, and, thereby, avoids difficult facts about the Irish situation such as the violent civil war in 1922 in which communities turned against each other. This is how my grandfather's fate was sealed, overnight, when he became "a traitor" to the Irish cause because he worked for the then British government.

Keith: I'd like to pick up some points about rebel songs, radicalism or being revolutionary, and activism.

Regarding the singing of Irish rebel songs—I'll admit, also with the benefit of hindsight and insight, that, alongside my thinking (in the form of a pretty consistent political analysis), my motivation at the time included a mixture of: a sense of belonging and wanting to belong—to and in a particular group and community; an identification with and identity as being on the Left (and, therefore on the side of the Angels!) and, yes, with that, was a certain collective righteousness; a rejection of "the British" and, with that, a dis-identification with being English (which lasted until my mid-30s, when I went to live in Italy and discovered my Englishness); and a certain yearning for the kind of solidarity which I saw in Irish, republican struggles and those of other oppressed groups. It felt good to be a comrade and an ally, and, for a certain period from the late 1970s through the 1980s, "the struggle" shaped a significant part of my life and activity. I'll also admit to the fact that I was—and, in many ways, still am—and idealist (and, to some extent, a Romantic). Although, since my early 20s, I have identified as a republican, there were (and still are) very few English republicans, and I suspect that this was also part of being drawn to Irish republicanism (as well as Scottish and Welsh republicanism), and, I have to say that, while I still remain seated for the British national anthem (which, of course is not about the nation but, rather, its hereditary monarch), I get hairs on the back of my neck when I hear Amhrán na bhFiann, Le Marseilles, Fratelli d'Italia, and other national anthems of Republics. So, when I sang and, from time to time, still sing republican/rebel songs, there's a lot to it—which doesn't mean to say that the singing or the song is nonetheless sincere.

Regarding "the revolution," one of the reviewers took issue with my comment about unequivocal and uncritical support for Irish republican and revolutionary demands, questioned what that meant, and commented that "if there is no real danger, there is no real revolution." I think it's good to be clear about this. Firstly, the keyword here is "demands." Big Flame did support the republican demand for a free and united Ireland and I stand by that. A critique of the history of the British conquest and partition of the island of Ireland (and many other geographical areas of the world) would support this. The means of achieving that end is another matter and not an easy one, which brings me to the second point: that of uncritical, *public* support. The point here is that any and every struggle against oppression is always criticised and undermined by the status quo, often with the full force of the state and sometimes with considerable brutality (here I thinking about slavery, the treatment of Suffragettes, the response of governments to independence movements, police reaction to demonstrators, etc.). In this context, such struggles need allies who are publically supportive; the last thing such struggles or movements need is for their allies to be equivocal or publicly critical. It's easy to critique liberation movements for their sexism, homophobia, and so forth. In its support for autonomous movements, however, Big Flame took the view that it/we would offer unconditional public support, and, through consistent and reliable solidarity work, would earn the right to have conversations in which we might raise questions of analysis, policy, strategy, and so on.

Regarding activism, while I think that Big Flame and other Left organisations were revolutionary in their analysis and ambition, and while some of us did come under the scrutiny of the British police's Special Branch, we were, arguably, in no great danger or, at least, we could choose whether to put ourselves in danger. Whether or not I was revolutionary, I was not *a* revolutionary, but I would claim to have been an activist. To me, this describes someone who is committed to a policy or action, usually through some form of campaigning, to bring about social/political change. I was and did, and, in some small ways, still do.

Helena: In his fascinating and knowledgeable account of the Irish Uprising R. F. Foster (2015) offers an analysis of the backgrounds and mentalities of those who ushered in the revolution. According to him, it was inspired by a multiplicity of intellectual motivations, from Connolly's socialist vision, to Pearce's fanatical connection with blood sacrifice and Catholicism, to the middle class Anglo Irish descendants who were affluent and had freedoms to play, and to be artistic, mystical, rebellious, and feminist—so from poets, socialists, artists, feminists, and religious believers, some of whom came from the aristocracy, sprang this Uprising which most of the ordinary people responded to with feelings such as "What are they on about?" and "For God's sake let's get on with it!" The contempt for "ordinary" people is shamefully apparent in Yeats' poem, "September 1913" in which he describes them as fumbling in "a greasy till" and adding the "halfpence to the pence" and "prayer to shivering prayer" (Yeats, 1996). Given this pre-revolutionary mix of hope and vision for diverse utopian futures, it is deeply ironic that instead, the revolution ushered in one of the most socially and politically conservative periods in Irish history. At the same time, as was pointed out by one of the reviewers, it is not so surprising, as many elements of Irish Republicanism had always been conservative, in the same way that Stalinism was conservative.

I recall my English mother, when we lived in Ireland for just four years in the 1950s, feeling deeply oppressed as a woman, mother, wife, and daughter. Her bitter memories included being told that "We don't hang the washing out on Sundays in our country" and "It's not the done thing to listen to the radio after 6.00 pm." She felt permanently chastised for behaving in "English" ways that a good Catholic Irish woman would never do, a judgement that also inferred that was "sluttish."

Another irony of the revolution was that in the pipeline had been a carefully worked out plan by people who genuinely cared for the ordinary Irish person, and about how best to proceed. This plan, the Redman Plan, would have involved the Irish nation taking complete control of their affairs, while still remaining under the banner of the UK, a banner which would have mitigated the influence of Catholicism, and allowed Protestant values to maintain and sustain the systems—to act as a modifying force so to speak. In the light of that I ask, what price Independence?—especially from today's perspective when we are all having to recognise, whether we like it or not, how interdependent we all are.

In Irish history, much has been made of the negative effect of Oliver Cromwell, and the British influence, in which they did, it is true, ban the Catholic religion and the Gaelic language. However, by 1914, the British had mellowed. Curiously, one of the things I learned recently was that the British introduced universal education before they did so in England. Another thing I learned was that in the planning of the Uprising, there was a big deal made of the Irish language but what they all had to come to terms with was that the English language was the one they all shared and so became the language of the revolution! In other words, pragmatism was privileged over Romanticism and sentiment, although the ideal of some Irish Garden of Eden, a return to an idyllic past, was very much part of the theme of the revolution.

The Redman Plan of course went out of the window in the wake of the Uprising because of the violent response by the British government. In executing the six leaders, they immediately set the scene for a revolution, the culmination of which offered the Irish government completely, and without equivocation, into the hands of Éamon De Valera and the Catholic church ushering in the death of any form of liberalism and has for a century, put the "ordinary" person into the clutches of people with the narrowest cultural and intellectual horizons. I recall in the 60s, my eternally creative Auntie Bridie explaining, in incomprehensible detail, why it was that she could take the contraceptive pill, not because she might wish to take control of her body, but because she had a "rare blood condition"!

While acknowledging De Valera as a hero who laid the foundation for an independent Ireland, Tim Pat Coogan (2015) made quite a damning assessment of De Valera's governance of Ireland, particularly in his co-creation of a political church-state monolith. Coogan's analysis resonates strongly with my recollections of my parents' experience. I recall sitting around the table at mealtimes, when we had already moved to the UK, and my parents being extremely critical of "Dev" as they referred to him, mocking his trenchant conservatism. He ruled Ireland with a fierce hand and mother seemed to hold him personally responsible for the severe social constrains which led to her needing literally to flee the country. Under his rule, the British were the "bad object" (discussed in more depth later) to such an extent that in the Second World War, he refused Churchill the use of the Irish ports in the fight against the Nazis, claiming it was because the English might use it as an opportunity to get a foot back onto Irish soil. This is a very contentious point, but, at the very least, it reflects the extent of the acrimonious relationship fostered by De Valera between Ireland and Britain.

And the Psychological

Keith: I was interested in your rediscovery of the Redmond Plan and the irony of pro-British Irish people being undermined by the reaction of the British state to the 1916 Irish Uprising, which, it appears, only had the effect of radicalizing ordinary Irish people into becoming even more anti-British! I wonder about the implications of a state coming into being and defining itself against another which sets up an external—and I think at some level internal—opposition.

I think about this in terms of impasse theory and, specifically, the interpersonal impasse, which I and Summers defined as: "the external manifestation of [an] intrapsychic impasse as split off parts of the self are projected onto the other. In this way the internal conflict gets enacted in an external relationship" (Tudor & Summers, 2014, p. 205)—in this application, between two peoples and nation states.

I've also been wondering about the psycho-political impact of a state being born against the background of what appears to have been a glorious and possibly inevitable failure, and rebellion. Reflecting on the Easter Uprising, Tóibín (2016) commented: "the power of the rebellion came from its symbolism as much as from its strategy." While I have a lot sympathy for rebellion and rebels, there is a cost to being in opposition, especially when this is done from a perspective of having a grievance. I think this is partly maintained by the reference to and use of heroes, and, predominantly, dead ones, such as, and perhaps most notably, Che Guevara.

I was also interested in your comments about the Catholic Church. I think there's another irony here which is that a new Republic, which, in many ways, epitomises the overthrowing of the old imperial(ist) parental/Parent authority (the British Crown), then uses and colludes with an institution (the Catholic Church) which, of course, enshrines a higher parental authority (God the Father). Some would argue, as Winnicott did about the British monarchy, that such authority, in this case the Church, provides a beneficent and stable parental authority. His analysis is a part of his theory of the use of an object (Winnicott, 1971) and, specifically, of a transitional object, that is, that the monarchy is a good object, which, unconsciously, the people would destroy; the fact that it survives both is reassuring and useful. Does the Irish Republican state provide a good—or good enough—object? I suspect not.

Helena: The personal is political and vice versa, so the saying going (Hanisch, 1970). You highlight exactly this process when you refer to "the irony of pro-British Irish people being undermined by the reaction of the British state." The execution of the leaders of the Uprising stimulated a nationalist fervour throughout the country in a way the rebels of the Uprising had failed to do. This could be a blueprint for how to initiate a revolution: alienate the people through a severe act of injustice!

When you wonder about "the implications of a state coming into being and defining itself against another which sets up an external ... opposition," again there feels to me to be a link between the personal and the political. The feelings toward the British are so personal in the Irish psyche. When I took my son, who has a London accent, over to Ireland in the 1980s, my unpleasant uncle, who had been in the Irish army, and who was seen to be the son of a traitor (as referred to above), sat in his armchair and sneeringly referred to my small, blond haired, little boy, as a "Brit," which sounded like a swear word. When I think about this now, I wonder if it was my uncle's way of trying to compensate for his lifelong experiences of feeling that he was not quite Irish enough, a strange legacy of the Uprising, with the unexpected consequences of turning Irish people, who worked legitimately for the incumbent government of the day, into "traitors." More recently, at a commemoration service in Dublin for the Uprising, it was reported that an Irish man turned around to a young woman present, who had a London accent, demanding that she account for her presence at the event. It turned out she was the great, great granddaughter of James Connolly! The roots of this bigotry can be traced back in part to some of the background of the Uprising. In Foster's (1915) book, I came across a story about the Irish Republican and Cumann na mBan activist, Mabel Fitzgerald, who was originally from a Presbyterian background in Ulster, but who was married to an Irish Republican. Infused with a zealotry, as converts so often are, she wrote to George Bernard Shaw to say that she was bringing up her son to adopt a hatred of England. According to Foster, Shaw replied that she was a wicked woman to fill her child's innocent soul with the burden of old hatred and rancor.

We may think about impasses from the perspective of object relations (Fairbairn, 1940), which describes the primitive psychological process of splitting in which the bad object is externalised onto something or someone, in this case the British, a process encouraged by De Valera. In my view, the object of the impasse has mistakenly been projected onto the "Brits" instead of the Catholic Church. Mind you, that could also be something to do with my projection! Although the younger generation (meaning the under 40s) are different. They are not so excised by anti-English sentiment. It seems to me that in taking back this projection they have become more resilient, stronger, more vibrant, with an increased sense of vital agency, as witnessed in May 2015 when the Irish voted by 62% or 38% in favour of gay marriage. This vote was not just about gay marriage. It was saying, we, the Irish are no longer in any shape or form to be governed or instructed by the Vatican. Goodbye! I spoke to many in Ireland during that time. The older ones were unsure, fearful, puzzled, and even ashamed. The younger ones were vibrant, clear, focused, and determined, with minds uncluttered by demonic threats of punishment for "sins" that may or may not have been committed suggesting a more mature integrated sense of self than their forefathers.

Of course neither the Uprising nor the vote for gay marriage happened in a vacuum. It would be absurd for instance to suggest that the vote for gay marriage happened because of a change in a nation's projection! In partic-ular, of course, the exposé of the role of the Catholic Church in child sexual abuse has played a vital part in the Irish turning away from the Vatican. There is a powerful video on YouTube showing the then Taoiseach, Enda Kenny, on exactly this subject (https://www.youtube.com/watch?v= hOQyl7ZpoH8). He almost sounds as though he is singing a rebel song: his tone so clear, his energy so vibrant, and his words so vital, as, in a direct reference to the ongoing child abuse investigations in Ireland, he warns the Vatican to stay out of Irish affairs. Of course, so many international developments influenced the gay vote, but it is beyond the scope of this rather personal set of reflections to offer an in-depth political analysis of every nuance and detail of how events have unfolded in Ireland.

This brings me onto your very interesting analysis of the role of the Catholic Church and the question of who occupies the role of the Parent ego state in our psyches. I was reassured recently by a colleague, who is an historian, explaining to me why British democracy is complex, old, and ingrained in such a way that we won't easily be destabilised. I should say that this was after the UK referendum on June 23, 2016, which determined that Britain should exit from the European Union which created a very divisive, and at times violent atmosphere in the country. The internalised Parent ego state is crucial, and you rightly point out Winnicott's analysis of the transitional object. Following on from this I began to think about ancient Ireland and its Celtic and pagan traditions before St. Patrick made his way over to the island and appropriated the customs and rituals, ideas, and beliefs to promote the Catholic way. What is Ireland's legitimate inherited Parent ego state? If no Catholic Church then what? The ancient ways linger in the psyche. In his book *How the Irish Saved Civilization,* Thomas Cahill (1995) traced the influence of the pagan and Christian scribes and how the Irish contributed to the liveliness and vitality associated with the Middle Ages. Although much criticised Cahill's book offers another story or myth about Ireland which serves to underlie the range and depth of the legacy of Irish-ness, whatever that may mean!

Keith: Yes, and of course, St. Patrick got rid of all those nasty snakes: a symbolic expulsion of feminine wisdom from the land, and an assertion of patriarchal Christianity, and, I would say, drawing on a critical reading of the Judeo-Christian creation myth, of speaking truth to power about the Tree of the Knowledge of Good and Evil.

Helena: I think the literary references are profoundly important too. They form an essential part of the narrative as do the rebel songs. In his poem "Easter 1916," for instance, Yeats reflects the ambivalence and puzzlement felt by many Irish people initially toward the Uprising. In the oxymoronic refrain, "A terrible beauty," Yeats captures this paradoxical experience of the Uprising. He also can't resist referring to Sean MacBride, the husband of his unrequited love, Maud Gonne, whom he couldn't stand, as a "vainglorious lout" (Yeats, 1996), yet who now has been transformed into one for whom he feels admiration—if a bit reluctantly!

I think there is much to be gained in seeing the revolution as a potent symbol as you mention in reference to Colm Tóibín. The rebel songs in particular reflect this symbolic significance, not so much of revolutionary fervour but of a passion for vitality, life, and a resistance to oppression. Rebel songs are like battle hymns, celebrating violent struggle, heroism, with the victim triumphing over their oppressor as in "The Dying Rebel": "The night was dark and the fight was over, | The moon shone down O'Connell Street." This song sets the scene and location of the Irish Uprising where the narrator meets dying men in the street: "I knew my son was too kind hearted, | I knew my son would never yield."

Tenderness and courage are linked, and later in the song, the son has gone "to heaven" as he is obviously a good Catholic! The songs refer to and historical event and create myth. The power of song has ancient roots, as Schenk (2011) put it: "Sung songs carry the paradoxical power of the Gods" (p.233). The way the song is sung of course is part of this and matters. Whoever has heard the mellifluous voice of Luke Kelly of the Dubliners sing "The Foggy Dew" cannot remain unchanged! Only in my view of course, but try it. His extraordinary energy, clear diction, fierce tone, surely carries a message from the Gods and yet listen too closely to the words and they disappoint in part because apparently only men who fought for Ireland and buried on Irish soil can be revered. Those brave Irish men who perished in Flanders and beyond fighting for the "dastardly" British in the First World War are merely cast aside as "traitors" who, therefore, cannot be mourned because they died in a foreign land. This narrative has at last found a more complex tone. In his book *A Long Long Way,* Sebastian Barry (2005) created a character called Willie Dunne who symbolises the Irish man/men who went to fight in the First World War. It is a heartbreaking story depicting the extraordinary bravery of the "ordinary" Irishman/men who put their lives on the line for what they thought was the "right" cause, only to face the madness of the trenches, and the status of a traitor at home. The Irish war heroes have only now been honoured this year in Glasnevin cemetery in Dublin as Ireland finally comes to terms with the complexities of its Anglo/Irish interconnectedness.

The rebel songs were perhaps also popular with some left wing groups in the UK during the 1970s in part because they also spoke of socialism:

> When Larkin came to Dublin,
> says he the poor have mighty weapons,
> to fight, to bring their oppressors down.
> (Plunkett, 1958)

The "weapons" referred to unions, and the ability to strike, as did the wonderful pean to James Connolly (composed by an unknown author), sung

with such passion, vigour, and conviction by Christy Moore (https://www.
youtube.com/watch?v=Z1tWwjWFmh8):

Where oh where is our James Connolly?
Where or where is that gallant man?
He's gone to organise the union,
That working men they might yet be free.

Romanticism, Modernism, and Postmodernism

Keith: As we've been corresponding, I've kept returning to Yeats' poem
about the Easter Uprising and the fact that it represented a shift in
him and his work—and perhaps the nation—from Romanticism to
Modernism. As Mlinko (2016) has pointed out, Yeats' early poems
feature his passion for Celtic mythology and Gaelic sagas, but in his
middle age, he became more attuned to the then current political
reality, later (in 1922), being appointed and serving as a Senator for
the Irish Free State. In 1913, he had published a poem, "September
1913," which commemorated his friend, John O'Leary, the Irish
nationalist, in which Yeats had written: "Romantic Ireland's dead
and gone, | It's with O'Leary in the grave." In many ways, this
prefigured his innovative poem about the Uprisings: "Easter 2016"
(Yeats, 1996). Mlinko (ibid) has summarized the significance of its
innovation, which "rested in Yeats's ability to preserve older
techniques that gave his verse its power—incantatory rhythm,
rhyme, symbolism, and allegory—while engaging frankly with the
interplay of personality, history, and politics of the present."

Apart from being an interesting and, I think, accurate reading of the poem
"Easter 1916," I wonder if this could be taken as a reading of the Easter
Rising itself. While the Rising was informed by Romantics (poets, linguists,
educationalists), the rebellion represented a break with Romanticism and
the establishment of a movement, which, within six years, had led to the
establishment of a modern and modernist Irish state. In this sense, I agree
with your critique of Four Green Fields. A couple of years ago, at a conference on Marxism, I had the good fortune to meet Eamonn McCann, the
Irish journalist and political activist from Derry, Northern Ireland/the
Six Counties. In the course of our conversation, we talked about Irish
rebel songs and he reported that, nowadays, Four Green Fields is hardly
ever sung. While I still think and feel that I want to honour rebels and
rebellion sometimes by singing rebel songs, I agree that all have a largely
symbolic function, and that it would be deeply ironic to romanticise a

rebellion against Romanticism! I think Anne Enright (2016) put it well when she wrote:

> All nations have founding myths. I suppose I would prefer to have a revolution in my country's past than a monarchy. I would prefer to move on from Catholic nationalism than from fascist dictatorship. But the truth is that local history has given way, in my lifetime, to global economics, and we have no good stories for this: no parades, no revolutions. The stories we tell ourselves about the past are not about politics. I mean they are not about fairness, about who has power and where the money goes. They contain a deeper madness.

As she—and you—has argued, we need to move on from Catholic nationalism, and, I would add, any other religious nationalism.

Of course, we now live in post-modern and more complex times:

> I was seven years old for the 50th anniversary of the Easter Rising, in 1966. The story had no complications. It was Ireland against England, good v bad, Irish Catholicism v paganism. And we won. We were the proof that we'd won, the boys and girls crammed into the classroom, learning the Proclamation of Independence, which was drafted by the leaders of the Rising, off by heart, from a tea towel that the teacher had pinned to the top of the blackboard, roaring the words out for Ireland. We didn't understand what we were shouting: "The Republic guarantees religious and civil liberty, equal rights and equal opportunities of all its citizens."

> Today, I love the complications. Many of the men in the GPO were actually English. I found that out only a few months ago. The children of Irish parents, they'd come over to Dublin from London, Manchester and Liverpool, to avoid conscription. The best named was Johnny "Blimey" O'Connor. (Doyle, 2016)

The vote for gay marriage marks not only a break with Rome (to coin a phrase) but also a rejection of ecclesiasticism, which, of course was a project of the Enlightenment. It thus marks another, quieter, but nonetheless glorious revolution, and a move(ment) into what we might refer to as a post-modern, post Catholic Ireland, and a much more free-thinking and empowered relationship with both Church and state. Moreover, the recent European Union (EU) referendum result in Northern Ireland (in which 56% of those who voted were in favour of remaining in the EU) raises the interesting prospect of that part of the now (dis)United Kingdom (UK) leaving the UK and joining Eire—or perhaps Scotland! While this outcome may be particularly fanciful—and, no doubt, Romantic(!)—it appears as if the old order is rapidly changing in ways in which we might not have previously dreamed or imagined.

Helena: However, I have come now to consider the other side of this passion and energy. In refusing and resisting oppression, one needs to find containment and thereby avoid the histrionics and superiority of Victimhood. Much has been made of the racism toward the Irish in England, yet I was interested to read, in her book *An Irish Navvy*, MacAmhlaigh's (1964) description of how many Irish people found that containment on British soil. In Britain, it became possible to earn a decent wage, raise children, have good educational opportunities, and free health care. The Irish in Britain were more detached and protected from the intrusion of the patriarchal tyranny of the Catholic Church.

In the late 20th century, the received wisdom was that Irish people emigrated for work; another, underlying narrative, which was not even entirely clear to themselves, is that they were also on the run from the conservatism of the Catholic Church, and, by most accounts, most found tolerance and acceptance in a Protestant Britain (MacAmhlaigh, 1964). In the 1950s, my father returned us all to Ireland, but left immediately because he said he could not find work, which was not entirely true: after four years my mother found the stifling conservatism so oppressive that she had a nervous breakdown and we returned to a more liberal Britain. One of my earliest observations about Protestants was their more casual and easy relatedness with their social and cultural environments.

And yet I still want to raise a flag for the rebel songs. I think now the feeling of them is what matters most. Their meaning now to me is to do with "home." Where is my heart? Where is my home? In his fascinating chapter on myth, Schenk (2011) describes how in Homer's *Odyssey*, "the uncertainty of home is illustrated in the role of song and storytelling," that the song "becomes a 'channel' for education, entertainment as well as a weapon of violent destruction" (p. 232). Maybe the song is a better channel for rage, for anger, for a wish to destroy. Maybe song is better than the gun—well no, not *maybe*, it *is*! Maybe the song is about a journey to find one's home in one's self. For me, the rebel songs are not just about the Irish struggle, they represent a gusty, powerful eloquence: a fierce energy, a life force that all those who seek self-agency recognise. I have witnessed it many times how often English people, without any political agenda, embraced and expressed a love of the rebel songs. I came to understand then that it wasn't just political: it was personal.

I have welcomed the opportunity to share some of my reflections on the Uprising. If there had not been an Uprising, I would never have been born, since my grandmother was engaged to a man who died on the streets in

1916, and subsequently met my grandfather. As Hillman (1996) pointed out in *The Soul's Code*, all births are random and it is a mystery how any of us get here! The legacy of the Uprising for me was that I was given life, though, with that, I also inherited a truly turbulent, distraught, paradoxical, and painful legacy, which Jung would have described as the "negre" we bring into therapy. Jung (1970/1990) used the alchemical metaphor to describe the analytic process of turning bad things into good things, the negre into "gold." Eigen (2006) describes how he works minute by minute with the psychic pain of trauma. Facing that pain has made me resilient and strong and enabled me to transform this harsh legacy into the gold dust, which means for me finding deep meaning and joy in my life and my work as a psychotherapist enabling me to reach into other peoples' hearts and minds, and to take part in their journey to find their true self, their home, their own way.

One final thought is based on another paradox described by Kiberd (1996), which is how the English and the Irish invented each other through projecting onto each other their own Shadow sides—which is good news for us all! The Irish can reclaim their potency and organisational capacities, and the English can own their lyricism and fondness for good hospitality.

Keith: Thank you, Helena. As someone who enjoys being a host, I'll settle for that, as well as the challenge of being (more) lyrical!

I have very much appreciated this dialogue. Of course, its origins go back to the late 1980s when we met as students on the transactional analysis psychotherapy training program at Metanoia, London, UK, and has been forged by much discussion and debate—and craic—over the years since then. I am also thinking that it represents a psychotherapy *of* politics (Totton, 2000), and a more dialogic and free-flowing form of the same psychopolitics that we represented in our collaboration on psychotherapy and citizenship (Tudor & Hargaden, 2002). I look forward to further and future dialogue, and collaboration.

REFLECTIONS

Keith Tudor is a well-known writer, psychotherapist, supervisor, and professor who now lives in New Zealand. Over the years, we have kept close contact and Keith has invited me on occasion to write for the many journals he has edited over the years. This chapter came about because he wanted us to write for the *Journal of Psychotherapy and Politics*. That is the surface understanding of how this came about but the origin of the chapter occurred in 1991 when Keith joined the training group I was in at the Metanoia institute. From the beginning, we made a political connection based on our former youthful involvement in left wing politics. Quite quickly it became clear to me that Keith and I formed an emotional bond around the subject of Ireland: during that dreadful era known as The Troubles with all the angst, pain, guilt, sacrifice, sorrows, rage, and at times the utter madness of what had happened and continued to happen on the blood-strewn streets of Belfast and beyond. I did not know his connection with Ireland at that time but I did feel a deep intimacy with Keith because I just knew that he "got it"; that he "got me," in all of mine and Ireland's utter complexity and "terrible beauty," which, in short, is the story of the Irish connection with the English and the English connection with the Irish! Although I have since diverted from my left wing political stance, we kept close collegial contact, which continued even when Keith went to New Zealand 13 years ago. As you can see from the chapter, my own political views became more complex, less binary, and more philosophical over the years. This chapter enabled me to reflect on my deep attachment to the Irish rebel song. I was only slightly surprised to find a multiplicity of meanings linked to defiance and rebellion and discover that at the core of myself, I will always own my own authority over ideology, religion, or any other type of coercive control. This is probably why I can appear quite difficult to some people when I refuse to conform, a type of coercion often used as a pressure to "belong." We have to belong to ourselves first and then we can belong anywhere as we choose.

Acknowledgment

We would like to thank both peer reviewers for their close reading and encouraging, informative—and challenging—comments, and to Sara Llelwellin for her comments on an earlier version of the chapter.

References

Allen, J.R. (2000). Biology and transactional analysis II: A status report neurode-velopment. *Transactional Analysis Journal, 30,* 260–269.

Aron, L. (2001). *A meeting of minds: Mutuality in psychoanalysis.* Hillsdale, NJ: The Analytic Press.

Aron, L. (2006). Colloquium Series: No. 9, 10/30/06 to 11/19/06 Topic: "Analytic Impasse and theThird: Clinical Implications of Intersubjectivity Theory"

Asay, T.P., & Lambert, M.J. (1999). The empirical case for the common factors in therapy: Quantitative finds. In M.A. Hubble, B.L. Duncan, & S.D. Miller (Eds.), *The heart and soul of change: What works in therapy* (pp. 33–56). Washington, DC: APA Press.

Bachelard, G. (1994). *The poetics of space.* Boston, MA: Beacon Press (Original work published, 1958).

Barry, S. (2005). *A long long way.* London, UK: Viking Press.

Bass, A. (2001). It takes one to know one; or, whose unconscious is it anyway? *Psychoanalytic Dialogues, 11*(5), 683–702. doi: 10.1080/10481881109348636

Bateman, A.W., & Tyrer, P. (2004). Psychological treatments for personality disorder. *Advances in Psychiatric Treatment, 10,* 378–388.

Bateson, G. (1972). *Steps to an ecology of mind.* New York: Ballantine.

Beebe, B., Jaffe, J., & Lachmann, F.M. (1992). A dyadic systems view of communication. In N.J. Skolnick & S.C. Warshaw (Eds.), *Relational psychoanalysis* (pp. 61–82). Hillsdale, NJ: The Analytic Press.

Benjamin, J. (1988). *The bonds of love.* New York: Pantheon Books.

Benjamin, J. (2002) 'Principles of Relational Psychoanalysis'. First biannual meeting of the International Association for Relational Psychoanalysis and Psychotherapy, New York.

Benjamin, J. (2004). Beyond doer and done to: An intersubjective view of thirdness. *Psychoanalytic Quarterly, 73,* 5–46.

Berne, E. (1961). *Transactional analysis in psychotherapy principles.* New York: Glove Press. (reprinted Guildford, CA: Shea Books, 1994). *principles.* Guildford.

Berne, E. (1964). *Games people play: The psychology of human relationships.* New York: Grove Press.

Berne, E. (1973). *Sex in human loving.* Harmondsworth: Penguin.

Berne, E. (1986). *Trasnactional analysis in psychotherapy: The classic handbook to its principles .* London: Condor.

Berne, E. (1994). *Principles of group treatment*. Menlo Park: Shea Books (Original work published 1966).

Bion, W.R. (1959). Attacks on linking. *The International Journal of Psycho-Analysis, 40*, 308–315.

Blackstone, P. (1993). The dynamic child: Integration of second-order structure, object relations, and self psy- chology. *Transactional Analysis Journal, 23*, 216–234.

Bollas, C. (1987). *The shadow of the object: Psychoanalysis of the unthought know*. New York, NY: Columbia University Press.

Bollas, C. (2000). *Hysteria*. London: Routledge.

Borges, J.L. (1923–1976). Obra Poetica. Emece. 2005.

Bowlby, J. (1958). The nature of the child's tie to his mother. *International Journal of Psycho-analysis, 39*, 350–373.

Brazelton, T.B., & Cramer, B.G. (1991). *The earliest relationship: Parents, infants and the drama of early attachment*. London: Karnac Books.

Brazelton, T.B., Tronick, E., Adamson, L., Als, H., &Wise, S. (1975). *Early mother-infant reciprocity [Ciba Foundation Symposium 33]*. London: Karnac Books.

Britton, R. (1989). The missing link: Parental sexuality in the Oedipus complex. In R. Britton, M. Feldman, Amsterdam: Elsevier.

Britton, R. (1998). *Belief and imagination: Explorations in psychoanalysis*. London: Routeldge.

Bromberg, P.M. (2006). *Awakening the dreamer: Clinical journeys*. Mahwah, NJ: The Analytic Press. *Chambers dictionary* (13th ed.) (2014). London, England: Chamber Harrap Publishers.

Bruner, J.S. (1977). Early social interaction and language acquisition. In H.R. Schaffer (Ed.), *Studies in mother-infant interaction*. London: Academic Press.

Bruner, J.S. (1981). Intention in the structure of action and interaction. In L.P. Lipsitt (Ed.). *Advances in infant research* (Vol. 1). NJ: Ablex.

Cahill, T. (1995). *How the Irish saved civilization*. London, UK: Stodder & Clark, B. (1991).

Chaasseguet-Smirgel, J. (1974). Perversion, idealisation and sublimation. *International Journal of Psycho-Analysis, 55*, 349–357.

Chodorow, N. (1978). *The reproduction of mothering*. Berkeley: University of California Press.

Clark, B. (1991). Empathic transactions in the deconfusion of the child ego state. *Transactional Analysis Journal, 21*, 92–98.

Clarkson, P. (1991). Through the looking glass: Explorations in transference and countertransference. *Transactional Analysis Journal, 21*, 99–107. doi: 10.1177/03 621537910210020n(2019)

Chambers dictionary (13th ed.). (2014). London: Chambers Harrap Publishers.

Coogan, T.P. (2015). *De Valera: Long fellow, long shadow*. London, UK: Cornerstone Arrow Books.

Cornell, W.F. (1988). Critique of script theory. *Trans actional Analysis Journal, 18*, 270–282.

Cornell, W.F., & Hargaden, H. (2005). *From transactions to relations*. London: Haddon Press.

Cornell W.F., & Hargaden, H. (Eds.). (2019). The evolution of a relational paradigm in transactional analysis: What's the relationship got to do with it? London:Routledge.

Damasio, A. (1999). *The feeling of what happens*. London: Heinemann.

Davies, J.M., & Frawley, M.G. (1992). Dissociative processes and transference-countertransference paradigms in the psychoanalytically oriented treatment of adult survivors of childhood sexual abuse. *Psychoanalytic Dialogues, 2*, 5–36.

Davies, P. and his team at the Centre for Research into Reading, Information and Linguistic Systems at the University of Liverpool (2010). Reading For Life. Oxford University.

Diamond, N., & Marrone, M. (2003). *Attachment and intersubjectivity*. London: Whurr Publishers.

Dimen, M. (2003). Sexuality and suffering, or the 'eeew!' factor IARPP (pp. 1–17), 19 May 2004.

Doyle, R. (2016, March 26). The Easter Rising 100 years on. *The Guardian*. Retrieved 25 July, 2016, from https:// www.theguardian.com/books/2016/mar/26/easter-rising-100-years-on-a-terrible-beauty-is-born.

Dylan, B. (1965). *Mr Tambourine Man*. Columbia, New York. Recorded at Columbia Studios, Hollywood.

Dylan, B. (1967). *Love is just a four letter*. Recorded at Columbia Studios, Hollywood

Eigen, M. (2007). *Feelings matter*. London: Karnac Books.

English, F. (1969). Episcript and the "hot potato" game. *Transactional Analysis Bulletin, 8*(32), 77–82.

English, F. (1976). Racketeering. *Transactional Analysis Journal, 6*, 78–81.

English, 1 F. (1969). *Transactional Analysis Bulletin, 8*(32), 77–82.

Enright, A. (2016, March 26). The Easter Rising 100 years on. *The Guardian*. Retrieved 25 July, 2016, from https://www.theguardian.com/books/2016/mar/26/easter-rising-100-years-on-a-terrible-beauty-is-born

Epstein, L., & Feiner, A.H. (1979). *Countertransference*. Northvale, NJ: Jason Aronson.

Erskine, R. (1991). Transference and transactions: Critiques from an intrapsychic and integrative perspective. *Transactional Analysis Journal, 21*, 63–76.

Erskine, R. (1993). Inquiry, attunement and involvement in the psychotherapy of dissociation. *Transactional Analysis Journal, 23*, 184–190.

Erskine, R. (1994). Shame and self-righteousness. *Transactional Analysis Journal, 24*, 86–102.

Erskine, R. (2001). Psychological function, relational needs, and transferential resolution: Psychotherapy of an obsession. *Transactional Analysis Journal, 31*(4), 220–226.

Erskine, R. (2008). Psychotherapy of unconscious experience. *Transactional Analysis Journal, 38*, 128–138.

Erskine, R.G. (2013). Relational group process: Developments in a transactional analysis model of group psychotherapy. *Transactional Analysis Journal, 43*, 262–275.

Erskine, R.G., & Trautmann, R.L. (1996). Methods of an integrative psychotherapy. *Transactional Analysis Journal, 26*, 316–328.

Erskine, Richard G., Moursund, Janet P., & Trautmann, Rebecca L. (1999). *Beyond empathy: A therapy of contact in relationship*. Philadelphia: Bruner/Mazel.

Fairbairn, R. (1952). Schizoid factors in the personality. In *Psycho-analytic studies of the personality* (pp. 3–27). London, UK: Routledge & Kegan Paul (Original work published 1940).

Farber, Sharon K. Becoming a telepathic tuning fork: Anomalous experience and the relational mind. *Anomalous Experience and the Relational Mind, Psychoanalytic Dialogues, 27*(6), 719–734. doi: 10.1080/10481885.2017.1379329

Feltham, C. (Ed.), *What's the good of counselling & psychotherapy?: The benefits explained.* Sage Publications Ltd.

Ferenczi, S. (1932). *The clinical diary of Sandor Ferenzi.* J. Dupont (Ed.). Cambridge, MA: Harvard University Press, 1988.

Fivas-Depeursinge, E. (1991). Documenting a time-bound, circular view of hierarchies: A microanalysis of parent-infant dyadic interaction. *Family Process, 30,* 101–120.

Fonagy, P., & Target, M. (1998). Mentalization and the changing aims of child psychoanalysis. *Psychoanalytic Dialogues, 8,* 87–114. doi: 10.1080/10481889809539235

Foster, R.F. (2015). *Vivid faces: The revolutionary generation in Ireland 1890–1923.* Harmondsworth, UK: Penguin Books.

Frawley-O'Dea, M.G. (1997). "Who's doing what to whom?" *Contemporary Psycho-Analysis, 33,* 5.

Freud, S. (1917). Mourning and melancholia, *Standard Edition, 14,* 237–258.

Freud, S. (1953). The interpretation of dreams. In J. Strachey (Ed. & Trans.), *The standard edition of the complete psychological works of Sigmund Freud* (Vols. 4–5) (Original work published 1899).

Freud, S. (1957). Mourning and melancholia. In J. Strachey (Ed. & Trans.), *The standard edition of the complete psychological works of Sigmund Freud* (Vol. 14, pp. 237–258). London: Hogarth Press (Original work published 1917).

Freud, S. in McGuire, W. (1974, pp. 239–231) The Freud/Jung Letters. Princeton University Press as referenced by Tansey, Michael J. (1994) Sexual Attraction and Phobic Dread in the Countertransference Psychoanalytic Dialogues, 4:2, pp. 130–152.

Freud, S. (1985). Totem and taboo. In J. Strachey (Ed. & Trans.), *The standard edition of the complete psychological works of Sigmund Freud* (Vol. VIII, pp. xii–162). London, UK: Hogarth Press.

Fromm, E. (1960). Psychoanalysis and Zen Buddhism. In D.T. Suzuki, E. Fromm, & R. DeMartino A. (2005). *Key ideas for a contemporary psychoanalysis: Misrecognition and recognition of the unconscious (A. Weller, Trans.). Hove, England: Routledge. (Eds.), Zen Buddhism and psychoanalysis.* New York: Harper & Row.

Gabbard, G.O. (1992). Commentary on "dissociative processes and transference-countertransference paradigms" by Jody Messler Davies and Mary Gale Frawley. *Psychoanalytic Dialogues, 2,* 37–47.

Gabbard, G.O. (1997). Nonsexual and sexual boundary violations between analyst and patient: A clinical perspective, Paper presented at Scientific Meeting of the British Psycho-Analytic Society, 5 November 1997, pp. 1–8.

Gerrard, J. (1999). Love in the time of psychotherapy erotic transference and countertransference: Clinical practice in psychotherapy. London: Routledge.

Gerson, S. (2004). The relational unconscious: A core element of intersubjectivity, thirdness, and clinical process. *Psychoanalytic Quarterly, 73*, 63–98.

Gerson, S. (2006). On analytic impasse and the third: Clinical implications of intersubjectivity theory (posting). In L. Aron (Ed.), and B. Reis & D. Shaw (Moderators), *Analytic Impasses and the Analytic Third. International Association fo Relational Psychoanalysis and psychotherapy*. Online Colloquium No. 9 www.iarpp.net/resource/colloquia/colloquium_9.html

Goldner, V. (1991). Toward a critical relational theory of gender. Psychoanalytic

Goulding, M. M., & Goulding, R. L. (1979). Changing lives through redecision therapy. New York. Grove Press.. *Power in the helping professions*. New York, NY: Spring Publications. Books.

Green, A. (2005). *Key ideas for a contemporary psychoanalysis: Misrecognition and recognition of the unconscious* (A. Weller, Trans.). Hove, England: Routledge.

Grossmark, R., & Wright, F. (2015). *The one and the many*. Routledge.

Guggenbuhl-Craig, A. (1971). *Power in the helping professions*. New York, NY: Spring Publications. HBooks.

Guntrip, H. (1962). The Schizoid compromise and psychotherapeutic stalemate. *British Journal of Medical Psychology, 35*, 273.

Hanisch, C. (2000). The personal is political. In B.A. Crow (Ed.), *Radical feminism: A documentary reader* (pp. 113–117). New York, NY: New York University Press (Original work published 1970).

Hargaden, (2019). Father where art thou? The significance of transgenerational trauma in a psychotherapy with Luke. *Transactional Analysis Journal, 49*(4), 248–262. doi: 10.1080/03621537.2019.1649933

Hargaden, H. (2001). There ain't no cure for love: The psychotherapy of an erotic transference. *Transactional Analysis Journal, 31*(4), 213–220.

Hargaden, H. (2004, 9 June). Two-chair work. Message posted to http://relationalta@topica.com (to access, see www.relationalta.co.uk).

Hargaden, H. (2010). When parting is not such sweet sorrow. In R.G. Erskine (Ed.), *Life scripts: A transactional analysis of unconscious relational patterns* (pp. 55–71, 249–272). London, England: Karnac Brunner/Routledge.

Hargaden, H. (2014). The role of boundaries and the third in relational group therapy. *Transactional Analysis Journal, 43*, 284–290. doi: 10.1177/0362153 713515178

Hargaden, H. (2016). The role of the imagination in n analysis of unconscious relatedness *Transactional Analysis Journal*, 2016, *46*(4), 311–321. doi: 10.1177/03 62153716662624

Hargaden, H., & Fenton, B. (2005). An Analysis of Nonverbal Transactions drawing on theories of Intersubjectivity. *Transactional Analysis Journal, 35*, 173–186.

Hargaden, H., & Sills C. (2001). Deconfusion of the child ego state: A relational perspective. *Transactional Analysis Journal, 31*(1), 55–70. doi: 10.1177/0362153701 03100107

Hargaden, H., & Sills, C. (2002). *Transactional analysis: A relational perspective*. London: Routledge.

Hargaden, H., & Tudor, K. (2016). The Irish uprising of Easter 1916: A psycho-political dialogue.

Haykin, M. (1980). Typecasting: The influence of early childhood experience upon the structure of the child ego state. *Transactional Analysis Journal*, 354–364.

Heaney, S. (2002). Finders Keepers: Selected Prose 1971–2001, Faber & Faber.

Hillman, J. (1996). *The soul's code*. London, UK: Bantam Books.

Hoffman, I. (1992). Some practical implications of a social-constructivist view of the psychoanalytic situation. *Psychoanalytic Dialogues*, *2*, 287–304.

Hoffman, I. (1998). Ritual and spontaneity in the psychoanalytic process. New Jersey: The Analytic Press.

Jorgenson, E.W., & Jorgenson, H.I. (1084). *Eric Berne: Master gamesman*. Grove Press.

Jung, C.G. (1978). *Man and his symbols*. London, England: Picador.

Jung, C.G. (1990). *The archetypes and the collective unconscious* (Vol. 9, part 1). London, UK: Routledge (Original work published 1970).

Karpman, S. (1968). Fairy tales and script drama analysis. *Transactional Analysis Bulletin*, *7*(26), 39–43.

Keats, J. (1817). Lewtter to brothers George and Tom.

Kiberd, D. (1996). *Inventing Ireland*. New York, NY: Vintage.

Kirschenbaum, H., & Henderson, V. (1990). *The Carl Rogers reader*. London: Constable and Company.

Klein, M. (1988). *Envy and gratitude and other works 1946–1963*. London: Virago Books (Original work published 1975).

Klein, M. (1986). *The selected Melanie Klein (1. Mitchell/Ed.)*. London: Peregrine Books.

Kohut, H. (1971). *The analysis of the self: A systematic approach to the psycho-analytic treatment of narcissistic personality disorder*. New York: International Universities Press.

Kohut, H. (1984). *How does analysis cure?* Chicago: University of Chicago Press.

Kraemer, S. (1999) 'Infant observation', *Tavistock Institute Videos*, London: BBC.

Kristever, J. (1980). *Desire in language: A semiotic approach to literature and art*. Oxford, England: Blackwell (Original work published 1969 in French).

Lacan, J. (1977). *Ecrits: A selection* (A. Sheridan, Trans.). New York, NY: Norton.

Leader, D. (2008). *The New Black*. London: Hamish Hamilton.

Leader, D. (2008). *The New Black: Mourning, melancholia, and depression*. London: Hamish Hamilton.

Lennon, J. (1970). *Mother. On John Lennon Plastic Ono Band (CD)*. United States: Apple Records.

Little, R. (2006). Treatment considerations when working with pathological narcissism. *Transactional Analysis Journal*, *36*(4), 303–317.

MacAmhlaigh, D. (1964). *An Irish Navvy: The diary of an exile*. London, UK: Routledge & Kegan Paul.

Makem, T. (1967). Four green fields. Retrieved, September 2016, from http://celtic-lyrics.com/lyrics/205.html

Mann, D. (1997). *Psychotherapy: An erotic relationship*. London: Routledge.

Mann, D. (ed.) (1999). *Oedipus and the unconscious erotic countertransference in erotic transference and countertransference: Clinical practice in psychotherapy*. London: Routledge.

Marion, J.-L. (1998). *Reduction and givenness: Investigations of Husserl, Heidegger, and phenomenology (studies in phenomenology and existential philosophy)* (T.A. Carlson, Trans.). Evanston, IL: Northwestern University Press.

Masson, J. (1988/1990). *Against therapy*. London: Fontana Paperbacks.

McGilchrist, I. (2009/2019). *The master and his emissary*. Yale University Press.

McLaughlin, J.T. (2005). *The healer's bent: Solitude and dialogue in the clinical encounter*. Hillsdale, NJ: Analytic Press.

Meier, C.A. (1995). *Personality*. Switzerland, Einsiedeln: Daimon (First published 1977 in German Walter-Verlag).

Menaker, E. (1995). *The freedom to inquire*. Northvale, NJ: Jason Aronson.

Miell, D., & Dallos, R. (1996). *Social interaction and personal relationships*. London: Sage.

Mitchell, S. (1988). *Relational concepts in psychoanalysis*. Massachusetts: Harvard Univesity Press.

Mitchell, S. (1993). *Hope and dread*. New York: Basic Books.

Mitchell, S.A. (1988). The intrapsychic and the interpersonal: Different theories, different domains, or historical artifacts. *Psychoanalytic Inquiries, 8*, 472–496.

Mitchell, S.A. (1997). *Influence and autonomy in psychoanalysis*. Hillsdale, NJ: The Analytic Press.

Mlinko (2016). William Butler Yeats: "Easter, 1916". How the conflict of a nation was captured by a politically reluctant poet. Retrieved 25 July, 2016, from https://www.poetryfoundation.org/resources/learning/core-poems/detail/43289#guide

Moiso, C. (1985). Ego states and transference. *Transactional Analysis Journal, 15*, 194–201. doi: 10.1177/036215378501500302

Moiso, C., & Novellino, M. (2000). An overview of the psychodynamic school of transactional analysis and its epistemological foundations. *Transactional Analysis*.

Morrison, B. (2001). Independent Newspaper, UK.

Morrisson, V. (1983). Inarticulate speech of the heart. Polydor, 839604-2. Instrumental and Song. On CD of same name.

Naiburg, S. (2015). *Structure and spontaneity in clinical prose*. New York, NY: Routledge.

Novak, E.T. (2015). Are games, enactments, and reenactments similar? No, yes, it depends. *Transactional Analysis Journal, 45*, 117–127.

Novellino, M. (1984). Self-analysis and countertransference. *Transactional Analysis Journal, 14*, 63–67.

Novellino, M. (1990). Unconscious communication and interpretation. *Transactional Analysis Journal, 20*, 168–172.

Oates, J. (1994). First relationships. In J. Oates (Ed.), *The foundations of child development* (pp. 259–298). Oxford: Blackwell/The Open University.

Ogden, T. (1982/1992). *Projective identification and psychotherapeutic technique*. London: Karnac Books.

Ogden, T. (1991). *The primitive edge of experience*. Northvale, NJ: Aronson.

Ogden, T. (1992). *Projective identification and psycho-therapeutic technique*. New York: Jason Aronson.

Ogden, T. (2004). The analytic third: Implications for psychoanalytic theory and technique. *The Psychoanalytic Quarterly*.

Ogden, T. (2004). On psychoanalytic writing. *International Journal of Psychoanalysis, 66*, 15–29.

Orange, D.M., Atwood, G.E., & Stolorow, R.D. (1997). *Working intersubjectively: Contextualism in psychoanaytic practice.* Hillsdale, NH: Analytic Press.

O'Shaughnessy, E. (Eds.), *The Oedipus complex today* (pp. 83–102). London: Karnac Books.

Pneuma. (2016). In *Wikipedia*. Retrieved from https://en.wikipedia.org/wiki/Pneuma

Rogers, A. (2008). *The unsayable: The hidden language of trauma.* New York, NY: Ballantine Books.

Rogers, C.R. (1967). *On becoming a person: A therapist's view of psychotherapy.* London: Constable & Constable (Original work published 1961).

Rustin, S. (2008, January 26). *The psychoanalyst Darian Leader says we've forgotten how to mourn, and that our understanding of relationships and our emotional life is 'catastrophic'. So, are you sitting comfortably?* London: The Guardian.

Rycroft, C. (1995). *A critical dictionary of psychoanalysis* (2nd ed.). London: Penguin.

Samuels, A. (1999). From sexual misconduct to social justice. In D. Mann (Ed.), *Erotica transference and countertransference: Clinical practice in psychotherapy.* London: Routledge.

Schaverin, J. (2015). *Boarding school syndrome: The psychological trauma of the 'privileged' child.* London, England: Routledge.

Schenk, R. (2011). Bed, bath and beyond: The journey that is not a journey/The home that is not a home – Psyche between home and homelessness in the Odyssey. In V.B. Rutter & T. Singer (Eds.), *Ancient Greece, modern psyche: Archetypes in the Sandler, J. (1993). On communication from patient to analyst: Not everything is projective identification. International Journal of Psycho-Analysis, 74, 1097–1107.* (pp. 221–247). London, UK: Routledge.

Schiff, L., Schiff, A. W., Mellor, K., Schiff, E., Schiff, S., Richman, D., Fishman, 1., Wolz, L., Fishman, C., & Momb, D. (1975). *Cathexis reader: Transactional analysis treatment of psychosis.* New York: Harper & Row.

Schinoda-Bolen, J. (1984). *Goddesses in everywoman.* New York, NY: Harper & Row.

Schore, A. (1994). *Affect regulation and the origin of self.* New Jersey: Lawrence Erlbaum Associates.

Schore, A.N. (2012). *Affect regulation and the repair of the self.* London, England: Norton (Original work published 2003).

Shakespeare, W. (1602). *Hamlet, in Bloom, 'The Invention of the Human', (1998).* Longman.

Shaw, D. (2014). *Traumatic narcissism: Relational systems of subjugation.* New York, NY: Routledge.

Shmukler, D. (1991). Transference and transactions: Perspectives from developmental theory. Object relations, and transformational process. *Transactional Analysis Journal, 21*, 127–135.

Sills, C. (1995, August). From ego states and transference to the concept ofsetting in transactional analysis: Reviewing the healing relationship. Panel presentation presented at the annual conference of the International Transactional Analysis Association, San Francisco.

Sills, C. (2001). The man with no name: A response to Hargaden and Erskine. *Transactional Analysis Journal, 31*(4), 227–232.

Slochower, J.A. (1996). *Holding and psychoanalysis: A relational perspective.* Hillsdale, NJ: The Analytic Press.

Stark, M. (1998). When the body meets the mind: What body psychotherapy can learn from psychoanalysis. Panel presentation at the First National Conference of the United States Association for Body Psychotherapy.

Stark, M. (2000). *Modes of therapeutic action.* Northvale, NJ: Jason Aronson.

Stern, D.N. (1985). *The interpersonal world of the infant: A view from psychoanalysis and developmental psy-chology.* New York: Basic Books.

Stern, D.N. (1993). Non-interpretive mechanisms in psychoanalytic therapy – The "something more" than interpretation. *International Journal of Psycho-Analysis. 79,* 903–921.

Stewart, I. (1992). *Eric Berne.* Sage Publications Ltd.

Stolorow, R. (1995). An intersubjective view of self psychology. *Psychoanalytic Dialogues, 5,* 393–400.

Stuthridge, J. (2012). Traversing the fault lines: Trauma and enactment. *Transactional Analysis Journal, 42,* 238–251.

Sullivan, H.S. (1953). *The interpersonal theory of psychiatry.* New York: Norton.

Tansey, Michael J. (1994). Sexual Attraction and Phobic Dread In the Countertransference *Psychoanalytic Dialogues, 4*(2), 130–152.

Thompson, C.M. (1964). The role of the analyst's personality in therapy. In M.R. Green (Ed.), *Interpersonal psychoanalysis.* New York: Basic Books (Original work published 1956).

Tóibín, C. (2016, March 26). The Easter rising 100 years on.*The Guardian.* Retrieved 25 July, 2016, from https://www.theguardian.com/books/2016/mar/26/easter-rising-100-years-on-a-terrible-beauty-is-born

Tolstoy, L. (1878/2003). Penguin Classics. Richard Pevear (Introduction, Translator).

Totton, N. (2000). *Psychotherapy and politics.* London, UK: Sage.

Trevarthen, C. (1979). Communication and co-operation in early infancy: A description of primary intersubjectivity. In M. Bullara (Ed.), *Before speech: The beginning of human communication.* London: Cambridge University Press.

Trevarthen, C. (1984). Emotions in infancy: Regulators of contacts and relationships with persons. In K. Scherer & P. Elkman (Eds.), *Approaches to emotions.* Hillsdale, NJ: Lawrence Erlbaum Associates.

Trevarthen, C. (1993). The functions of emotions in early infant communication and development. In J. Nadel & L. Camioni (Eds.), *New perspectives in early com-municative development.* London: Routledge.

Tudor, K., & Hargaden, H. (2002). The couch and the ballot box: The contribution and potential of psychotherapy? *The benefits explained* (pp. 156–178). London, UK: Sage.

Tudor, K., & Summers, G. (2014). *Co-creative transactional analysis: Papers, dialogues, responses, and developments.* London, UK: Karnac Books.

Vygotsky, L.S. (1962). *Thought and language* (E. Haufmann & G. Vakar, Eds. & Trans.). Cambridge, MA: MIT Press.

Vygotsky, L.S. (1978). *Mind in society: The development of higher psychological processes* (M. Cole, V. John-Steiner, S. Scribnerand, & E. Souberman, Eds.). Cambridge, MA: Harvard University Press.

Vygotsky, L.S. (1988). The genesis of higher mental functions. In K. Richardson & S. Sheldon (Eds.), *Cognitive development to adolescence*. Hove: Lawrence Erlbaum Associates.

Watzlawick, P. (1963). A review of the double-bind theory. *Family Process, 2*(1), 132–153.

William Butler Nevin, D. (Ed.) (2006). *James Larkin: Lion of the fold*. Dublin, Ireland: Gill & Macmillan.

Williams, P. (2007). Contribution made on 17/5/2007: IARPP-Colloquium Series: No. 10, 5/14/07 to 5/28/07 Topic: *"When the Frame Doesn't Fit the Picture"* Author: Anthony Bass. Moderators: Bruce Reis and Daniel Shaw.

Winnicott, D.W. (1949). Hate in the countertransference. *International Journal of Psycho-Analysis, 30*, 69–74.

Winnicott, D.W. (1953). Transitional objects and transitional phenomena. *International Journal of Psycho-Analysis, 34*, 89–97.

Winnicott, D.W. (1960). *The maturational processes and the facilitating environment: Studies in the theory o f emotional development*. London: Hogarth Press.

Winnicott, D.W. (1984). The theory of the parent-infant relationship. In *The maturational process and the facilitating environment* (pp. 37–55). London, UK: Karnac (Original work published 1965).

Winnicott, D.W. (1985). *The maturational processes and the facilitating environment*. London: Hogarth Press.

Winnicott, D.W. (1986). The place of the monarchy. In C. Winnicott (Ed.), *Home is where we start from*. Harmondsworth, UK: Penguin (Original work published 1970).

Yeats, W.B. (1996). In R.J. Finneran (Ed.), *The collected poems of W. B. Yeats*. New York, NY: Scribner.

Yehuda, R., Engel, S.M., Brand, S.R., Seckl, J., Marcus, S.M., & Berkowitz, G.S. (2005). Transgenerational effects of posttraumatic stress disorder in babies of mothers exposed to the World Trade Center attacks during pregnancy. *Journal of Clinical Endocrinology & Metabolism, 90*(7), 4115–4118. doi: 10.1210/jc.2005-0550

Yehuda, R., Daskalakis, N.P., Lehmer, A., Desarnaud, F., Bader, H.N., Makotkine I., ... Meaney, M.J. (2014). Influences of maternal and paternal PTSD on epigenetic regulation of the gluco-corticoid receptor gene in holocaust survivor offspring. *American Journal of Psychiatry, 171*(8), 872–880. doi: 10.1176/appi.ajp.2014.13121571

Zeitlin, A., & Secunda, S. (Writers). (mid-1950s). Donna Donna (A. Kevess & T. Schwartz, Trans.). (Original published 1941 in Yiddish):Yeats, W. B. (1996). In R. J. Finneran (Ed.).

Index

Note: Page numbers in *italics* refer to figures

For Product Safety Concerns and Information please contact our EU
representative GPSR@taylorandfrancis.com
Taylor & Francis Verlag GmbH, Kaufingerstraße 24, 80331 München, Germany

9 781032 266220